THE
ENERGY
of
EVERYTHING

THE
ENERGY
of
EVERYTHING

REDISCOVERING VITALITY THROUGH QUANTUM WELLNESS

Philipp S. von Holtzendorff-Fehling

Published by Best Seller Publishing®, St. Augustine, FL
Best Seller Publishing® is a registered trademark.
Printed in the United States of America.

ISBN: 9781969338694

This publication is designed to provide accurate and authoritative information with regard to the subject matter covered. It is sold with the understanding that the publisher is not engaged in rendering legal, accounting, or other professional advice. If legal advice or other expert assistance is required, the services of a competent professional should be sought. The opinions expressed by the author in this book are not endorsed by Best Seller Publishing® and are the sole responsibility of the author rendering the opinion.

For more information, please write:
Best Seller Publishing®
1775 US-1 #1070
St. Augustine, FL 32084
or call 1 (626) 765-9750
Visit us online at: www.BestSellerPublishing.org

Disclaimer

The terms healing or healer may mean many things to many people. In a traditional sense, which fits nicely with today's approaches to support general wellness, healing refers to the release of blocked energy and the orchestration of its flow. This flow of energy, called by different names in different cultures, is needed on one level so that the physical happenings of the body can function harmoniously on another level. The intersection between the flow and orchestration of energy and the functioning of physical systems is a fascinating space for exploration of body systems in various states of function. However, while those physical systems may be described in terms of health or disease by today's physicians and society generally, please understand that use of the terms healing or healer in this book is intended to be viewed exclusively in reference to the release and orchestration of what is happening on the energetic level.

In this book, I choose to embrace and communicate in language that is consistent with a traditional view of energetic chakras being connected with and manifest in the physical body and its functions. This exploration and use of language to describe a traditional construct and viewpoint should not be construed as the presentation of a substitute for medical intervention that may be needed to treat or prevent disease.

The author does not recommend or endorse any specific tests, physicians, procedures, opinions or other information that may be mentioned in this book. Statements made in this book have not been evaluated by the Food and Drug Administration (FDA), the EFSA, or any other government derivatives thereof. The content, tools, and methods mentioned or described in this book are not intended to diagnose, treat, cure, or prevent any disease or health condition.

Dedication

To the infinite intelligence that flows through all of life—
the source of energy, frequency, and consciousness from which
we come, which we are made of, and to which we return.
May this work serve as a reminder that healing, harmony, and
limitless potential are not outside of us
but within us—always.
And to every soul ready to remember who they truly are—
this is for you.

The Energy of Everything

In a world awash with health hacks and surface-level wellness trends, this book is a breath of fresh, quantum-charged air. Philipp von Holtzendorff-Fehling doesn't just speak about energy—he embodies it. Blending ancient wisdom with modern science, he reveals that quantum wellness isn't a concept to study, but a state to live. This is more than a book—it's a transmission. A master key for anyone ready to cut through the noise and reclaim their energetic sovereignty.

—Luke Storey, Consciousness Explorer,
Host of *The Life Stylist Podcast*

As a doctor rooted in both Eastern medicine and modern functional science, I rarely encounter a book that so powerfully unites energy, healing, and performance. Philipp von Holtzendorff-Fehling offers a profound yet practical guide to quantum wellness—one that aligns deeply with traditional wisdom and the needs of today's high-performing individuals. I'll be recommending this to patients, athletes, and fellow practitioners.

—Dr. Jyun Shimizu, PhD Integrative
Medicine, Doctor of Acupuncture

This book is a powerful invitation to return to the essence of who we are. Philipp masterfully bridges science, ancient wisdom, and practical insight, offering a road map to vitality and our infinite healing potential. As a functional medicine practitioner, I deeply appreciate how his work uplifts and complements the healing journey in ways that go far beyond the physical realm.

—Dr. Brooke Stuart, Functional Medicine
Doctor & Founder of Let Go & Grow®

I've always been searching for harmony between mind, body, and soul. The life of a fighter has offered me the opportunity to intensify this search. Only when you live in harmony can you fully compete. Philipp's book is groundbreaking. It opens the door to a deeper level of human potential—something every athlete, healer, and conscious person should explore. It has been an essential part of my success so far.

—Natalie Zimmermann, two-time world boxing
champion and high-performance trainer

Foreword

As a quantum-level therapist and scientist with deep roots in consciousness architecture and frequency medicine, I keep an eye on works that can translate the invisible into the embodied. Philipp von Holtzendorff-Fehling has done precisely that.

This book is not simply a read—it's a field of coherence. A living bridge between quantum physics and human transformation, it carries the rare ability to marry scientific rigor with the vibrational essence of all. It doesn't dilute complexity, nor does it mystify the energetic—it harmonizes them.

With every page, the reader is invited into direct resonance with the Original Code—the deep intelligence that underlies all healing. It doesn't preach methods; it awakens memory. This is a quantum instrument for realignment, restoration, and conscious evolution.

A powerful contribution to the emerging era of frequency-based healing that is essentially becoming the Future of Medicine. A transmission for those ready to embody the future now.

With quantum respect,

Dr. Nataliya Storozhylova, 2x PhD, ex-Mindvalley, Pioneer in Quantum-Level Biohacking & Consciousness-Based Healthcare & Vibrational Medicine

Table of Contents

Section 1:
Where the Past,
Present, and
Future Meet

1
The Past and Present

"The natural healing force within each one of
us is the greatest force in getting well."
—Hippocrates

When we think about healing, it's easy to dismiss the contributions of the great civilizations that preceded modern society.

If they didn't have the scientific knowledge or technology that we possess today, how could they possibly know anything about healing?

There's a reason this chapter opens with a quote from Hippocrates. He's known as the "Father of Medicine," and in many countries, newly-minted doctors still take what's known as the Hippocratic Oath, named for him. The truth is, Hippocrates was not blessed with modern technology, but he was blessed with an astute mind, a keen ability for observation, and the courage to explore the wondrous properties of the human body.

Hippocrates's theory of Four Humors—Blood, Phlegm, Yellow Bile, and Black Bile—that aligned to the four elements—air, water, fire, and earth, respectively—became the basis for early Western medicine. Hippocrates believed that through achieving and maintaining balance between the Four Humors, people would stay in good health; any imbalance would manifest as a symptom of illness.

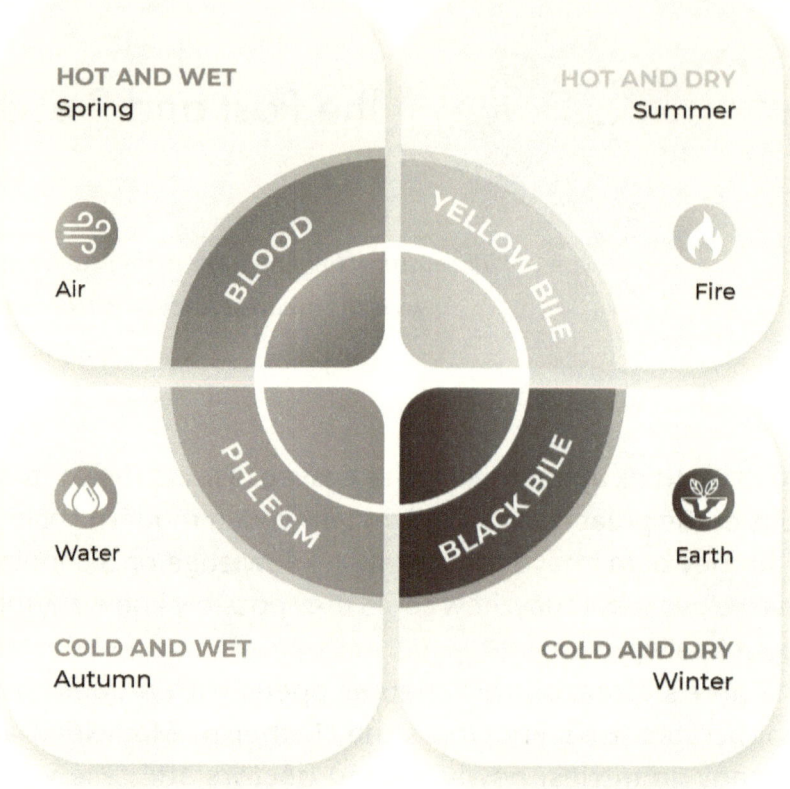

HOT AND WET
Spring

Air

HOT AND DRY
Summer

Fire

BLOOD

YELLOW BILE

PHLEGM

BLACK BILE

Water

Earth

COLD AND WET
Autumn

COLD AND DRY
Winter

Hippocrates believed that the Four Humors aligned to natural elements and human health.

A MIX OF BELIEF AND MEDICAL PRECURSORS

This is not to say that Hippocrates's contributions weren't valuable, but attempting to understand his contributions to medicine means putting him in the context of his time. Keep in mind that ancient Greece during the Classical Era was home to an unprecedented explosion of intellectual thinking. With the genius of Socrates, Plato, Aristotle, and others all working together, ethics, politics, metaphysics, and aesthetics came alive.

In such a milieu, it's no surprise that medicine saw great advancement as well. Hippocrates brought a rational view to medicine, rejecting the religious idea that illness was a punishment for wickedness and suggesting instead that disease had natural causes.

The Four Humors was a revolutionary idea and a step toward understanding the body in a systematic way. Blood, associated with air, was considered a hot and wet substance in charge of vitality and spirit, while phlegm, associated with water, was considered a cold and wet substance in charge of both the emotions and the functioning of respiration.

Meanwhile, yellow bile, associated with fire, was considered a hot and dry substance in charge of digestive functions and liver health. Black bile, associated with earth, was considered a cold and dry substance in charge of melancholy and the health of the spleen. Physicians were encouraged to think of the body in its environment, which is the uniquely holistic approach that we see in so many approaches to complementary therapies today.

Hippocrates also emphasized the importance of diet, exercise, and lifestyle for health and disease prevention. Although his advice comes laden with the language of the Four Humors, it is in many ways identical to what we hear today. If you break it down, he promoted a measured approach to everything, including healthy eating and regular physical activity.

Moreover, his insistence that Hippocratic physicians should treat the sick according to the best of their ability, and above all, do no harm, holds a powerful legacy in the form of the Hippocratic Oath, a profound ethical touchstone for any conscientious physician.

Using the powerful words of Hippocrates as a guide, it is easy to see how ancient forms of healing were neither superstitious nor outdated. Instead, they embody an essential shamanism so fundamental to human experience that it is the basis for every form of Western medicine the foundations of which share its principles. If we were to integrate these approaches with modern science, we could formulate a new health model that recognizes the power the body has to heal itself.

Nevertheless, for the true origins of healing, we need to look even further back in time to the ancient Egyptians and the Indigenous peoples of the American continents.

Healing techniques also evolved in the Chinese dynastic era and on the Indian subcontinent long before "modern" medical practices came into existence. Let's take a look at the connection between ancient healing techniques, which bear global similarities in their holistic mix of beliefs, ties to nature, and precursors to modern scientific findings.

Indigenous Healing Practices

Indigenous cultures in North, Central, and South America used a combination of herb-based remedies along with ceremonies and rituals that connected them with nature and the spirit world. While the plants and herbs varied greatly between regions, there is a common thread of finding balance and harmony between the body, nature, and the unseen among native tribes and cultures throughout the Americas.

In First Nation communities, healing practices often involve group sessions, where people share personal stories and experiences in a circle, passing a "talking stick" around. This process promotes healing and self-confidence. Emotions are considered central to being human and for tuning in to spiritual and relational responsibilities.

Emotion-focused healing ceremonies and rituals include the use of sweat lodges (or "purification lodges"), in which energy, emotions, and physical blockages are cleansed and released through the human body. A sweat lodge is a small, enclosed structure, in which individuals sit in a dark, steam-filled environment where stones have been heated.

The healing circle usually consists of an elder, leader, or traditional First Nation shamanologist who is knowledgeable about the local history, culture, and ceremonies. In sweat lodge healing ceremonies, elders and clan mothers may beat on drums and call upon ancestors, generators, and spirits through chanting. The use of sacred herbs such as sage, cedar, and sweetgrass are often used to cleanse and protect the energy of the patients.

Traditional healers in Native American cultures view healing as the responsibility of the patient, with healers serving as facilitators and counselors. They use stories, humor, music, tobacco, smudging, and ceremonies to bring healing energies into the space and focus their effects.

Smudging involves the heartfelt burning of herbs such as sage, cedar, and so on to clear off bad energy and restore order. Indigenous healers still use these 1,000-year-old methods alongside modern medicine today. For native cultures, healing is an all-encompassing outreach to engage, and thereafter make well, the whole person's mind, body, and spirit.

For native cultures, healing was and is a holistic endeavor. Rituals, prayers, and meditation were often integral to the process of healing, thought to bring the person being healed closer to nature and the spirit realm.

In Australian Indigenous culture, the traditional medicine practice (TMP) of the Aboriginal and Torres Strait Islander peoples includes the use of healers, healing songs, and bush medicines. Traditional healers have extensive knowledge passed down through generations and use plants for healing and preventing diseases. For example, they make use of tea tree oil, which has anti-inflammatory and antimicrobial properties and is widely used in the region. It originates from the Melaleuca alternifolia tree, native to New South Wales in eastern Australia. Healing songs called "songlines" are believed to contain the power that aids the person seeking healing to connect to the land and their ancestral spirit, guiding them through their physical and spiritual journeys.

These practices emphasize the interdependence of all life and place great importance on preserving balance within the person as well as with the natural surroundings. They carry forward the wisdom of Indigenous ancestors into a world that could still benefit from their advice.

Ancient Egyptian Beliefs and Methodologies

The healing practices of the ancient Egyptians bear a striking resemblance to Indigenous and First Nation healing practices despite developing on the other side of the world. Being a polytheistic culture also meant that the ancient Egyptians had temples dedicated to Imhotep, the god of healing, where people could come to receive treatment from priests who practiced healing.

Ancient Egyptian healing techniques were also quite holistic. They involved prayers, meditation, and medicinal treatments made from herbs and other natural materials. Treatments covered physical, spiritual, and emotional maladies and integrated prayers and meditation as part of the process.

Medicinal treatments included root extracts, resins, gums, and remedies made from herbs and other natural materials.

Ancient Egyptian healers even had official medical texts such as the Ebers papyrus, one of the oldest known medical documents, containing hundreds of remedies and prescriptions for a wide range of ailments. This extensive pharmacopoeia shows how sophisticated the Egyptians were in their understanding of natural, plant-based medicine. It included remedies for a wide variety of acute and chronic diseases including poisoning, ulcers, hemorrhoids, skin lesions, and eye infections.

The Egyptians also believed in the beneficial effects of protective objects, especially talismans and amulets. These items could protect the bearer from illness and excise evil spirits. They were often inscribed with spells and made of precious and semiprecious stones and metals. The forces were said to be drawn from the creator gods of heaven and imbued into the object, so its mere possession provided healing and protection.

Balance and harmony (are you sensing a theme here?) were also considered critical facets of healing in ancient Egypt. They called this life force Ma'at, and any imbalance or disruption in Ma'at could result in illness. Again, a holistic approach to healing involving the mind, body, and spirit formed the foundation of medicine for ancient Egyptians.

This integrative approach is also evident in their funerary practices. The art of mummification ensured that the body remained whole for the afterlife. Healing rituals, spells, and incantations were performed on the body to cleanse it of the deceased person's faults and sins. Disease was believed to be caused by evil spirits, so the spells were designed to expel these spirits and enhance the protective power of the amulets placed all over the body.

In short, the ancient Egyptian approach to healing was a complex practice that encompassed their religious beliefs as well as their mystical understanding of harmony and balance, and it served both therapeutic and social needs. Looking back at this rich legacy of advanced medicine and holistic healing makes it easy to see the interconnectedness of health practices through time.

The Indian Subcontinent and the Rise of Ayurveda

Another one of the world's oldest medical practices, *Ayurveda*, came to life on the Indian subcontinent in or around the sixth century BCE. The term *Ayurveda* comes from the Sanskrit words *ayur* and *veda*, meaning life and science.

Ayurveda bases its principles on three fundamental energies, or *doshas*, that correspond with the body's physical and psychological functions. Every person possesses their own individual, unique combination of these three energies, and to be healthy, the three must remain in balance. One's *prakriti*, or unique makeup, can help that person make lifestyle and dietary choices that keep their *doshas* in harmony.

Ayurveda is also based on a holistic approach to maintaining the balance of the five elements—earth, fire, air, water, and ether—which combine into the *doshas*. To do this, Ayurveda practitioners help people craft lifestyles of routine, diet, herbal medicine, yoga and meditation, and detoxification to keep their *doshas* in balance. It's a peaceful, whole-person approach to finding and maintaining health based on an individual's physical, emotional, and spiritual needs. Modern Ayurveda practitioners use a combination of ancient teachings and philosophies and current healthcare guidelines and treatments.

The Origins and Practices of Traditional Chinese Medicine (TCM)

The last ancient healing practice we'll explore in this opening chapter is traditional Chinese medicine, or TCM. This practice, which has evolved over thousands of years, is based on the concept of life force, or *Qi*, that flows through the body's energy pathways. The balance of Qi is thought to be necessary for good health, and imbalance leads to illness. To achieve optimal health, one's Yin and Yang, which are the opposing forces of Qi, must remain in harmony.

TCM also incorporates natural elements. Here, those elements are wood, fire, metal, water, and earth, which are each associated with specific emotions or internal organs. To keep a balance between the elements and Qi, practices like acupuncture, cupping, herbal medicine, and gentle exercises like Tai Chi and Qigong are employed alone or in carefully prescribed combinations. TCM also puts an emphasis on a balanced diet and good nutrition to naturally ward off illness. This holistic approach to maintaining health has endured since the early days of dynastic China and is still in use today in conjunction with modern medicine.

HOW ENERGIES AND FREQUENCIES FIT WITH HEALING PAST AND PRESENT

If there is one thing to be learned from these separate but similar ancient health practices, it's that natural energies are healing tools. Today, we know that everything in the universe, ourselves included, has its own energy. We and the matter that surrounds us vibrate at a particular frequency. Technology now allows us, up to a point, to measure that energy and frequency, as well as their effects. This is strong evidence to imply that, while they may have lacked the instrumentation, shamans and other healers were operating on the same principles we can now verify.

Pre-scientific practitioners around the world observed the workings of the natural world around them and collected their observations about energy flow in living things and in the greater order of the universe. Certainly, they did not refer to that energy as we, in the here and now, would; but whatever the name, practices such as acupuncture, herbal medicine, and spiritual healing rituals are all modalities that were developed for the same purpose.

They are all based on the manipulation of unidentified but detectable and extraordinary forces to gain wellness through the energy system already inherent in the human body. This breakthrough has been supported by technology that can spot and measure the myriad ways energy impacts us and our human biology. For example, MRI machines, EEGs, and similar technologies register and translate electrical impulses and fields in our bodies—proving what many ancient techniques tapped into concerning energy and frequency.

Technology, of course, also plays a role in the seemingly increasing amount of energy that is emitted throughout the world. I want to remind readers of the Law of Conservation of Energy, which states that energy cannot be created or destroyed; it can only be transferred from one form to another.

How can we account for the energy being drawn on and emitted by electronic devices and other technology? Through the Law of Conservation of Energy, we know that energy must be coming from somewhere. The source is—wait for it—organic matter, and that includes us!

With this in mind, we return to a central point about the modern environment: The amount of electromagnetic forces being generated by our technology is unparalleled in human history. Cell phones, Wi-Fi, microwaves, and all other electronics are constantly sending EMFs into the world. As we know, the body needs to be in a state of energy balance to be healthy.

Perhaps Atreya, the father of Ayurveda, could intuitively know how to balance the body with natural flows of energy by virtue of living in the natural world. Unfortunately, today we must take active measures to prevent interference from EMFs if we want to protect our health. If we were ancient medical practitioners or healers, we'd be scrambling to find a way to rebalance our life forces from the assault by microwaves, cellular signals, and electromagnetic forces that constantly bombard us.

So what can we do as modern humans? How can we take back our life forces?

Modern energy management tools include mindfulness and meditation, yoga, and Tai Chi or Qigong, interventions that traditionally built communities for millennia by strengthening our own magnetic force and connection to energy fields, or by promoting grounding, a.k.a. earthing. Earthing, which is contact with the earth, is one of the simplest interventions to neutralize EMFs and reconnect us with the earth's energy—it's the most ancient solution of all.

What's more, the technologies themselves can be harnessed to our benefit. Devices that shelter us from the effects of EMFs, such as EMF shields and harmonizers, protect the biofield, while biofeedback and neurofeedback technologies provide real-time information on physiological status. These technologies can enable us to make immediate adjustments to restore homeostasis and health.

As we live and work in an electromagnetic environment filled with sensory inputs from technology, we can also draw from both ancient wisdom and modern innovations to maintain and restore energy balance when it is disturbed. Marrying the wisdoms of the past with the tools of the present can help to bring about a convergence between health and well-being. Let's explore that idea in the next chapter.

References

1. Attewell, G. (2007). "Refiguring Unani Tibb: Plural Healing in Late Colonial India." *Social History of Medicine*, 20(1), 77–96.
2. Barnes, L. L., & Sered, S. S. (2005). *Religion and Healing in America*. Oxford: Oxford University Press.
3. Ebers papyrus. (n.d.). In Encyclopaedia Britannica. Retrieved from https://www.britannica.com/topic/Ebers-papyrus.
4. Elkin, A. P. (1993). *Aboriginal Men of High Degree*. St. Lucia: University of Queensland Press.
5. First Nations Health Authority. (n.d.). "Traditional Healing." https://www.fnha.ca/wellness/wellness-for-first-nations/traditional-wellness/traditional-healing/traditional-healing.
6. Hanson, A. E. (n.d.). "Hippocrates: The 'Great Miracle' in Medicine." *Medicina Antiqua,* University College London. https://www.ucl.ac.uk/~ucgajpd/medicina%20antiqua/sa_hippint.html
7. Jouanna, J. (1999). *Hippocrates*. Baltimore: Johns Hopkins University Press.
8. Kirmayer, L. J., & Valaskakis, G. G. (2009). *Healing Traditions: The Mental Health of Aboriginal Peoples in Canada*. Vancouver: UBC Press.
9. National Center for Complementary and Integrative Health. (2021). "Traditional Chinese Medicine: What You Need To Know." https://www.nccih.nih.gov/health/traditional-chinese-medicine-what-you-need-to-know.

10. Nunn, J. F. (1996). *Ancient Egyptian Medicine*. London: British Museum Press.
11. Nutton, V. (2004). *Ancient Medicine*. London: Routledge.
12. Pitchford, P. (2002). *Healing with Whole Foods: Asian Traditions and Modern Nutrition*. Berkeley: North Atlantic Books.
13. Unschuld, P. U. (1985). *Medicine in China: A History of Ideas*. Berkeley: University of California Press.
14. Wilcox, R. A., & Whitham, E. M. (2003). "The symbol of modern medicine: Why one snake is more than two." *Annals of Internal Medicine*, 138(8), 673–677.
15. Wujastyk, D. (2003). *The Roots of Ayurveda: Selections from Sanskrit Medical Writings*. London: Penguin Books.

2
Where the Future Meets ...

"As cities grow and technology takes over the world, belief and imagination fade away ... and so do we."
—Julie Kagawa

Before we go any further, I want to point out that technology is not an enemy. Neither are most of the people who create it. Railing against technology as a whole is not the point of this book. We need to be mindful of generalizing the term *technology* and making a blanket statement that all digital, electronic, or otherwise nonorganic devices will be the downfall of society. That's not what we're here to discuss.

Thanks to technology, we have the ability to improve and save lives. It has improved processes in medicine and other areas. It has also given us the ability to communicate across the earth instantly and at all times.

We've also seen how technology can improve our lives in ways we never could have imagined before they were invented. But so, too, come the pitfalls. There's the issue of excessive dependence on devices and the privacy of personal information; there's e-waste and the environmental burden of consumerism. The solution is to use technology in a way that complements our natural skills rather than undermining them. But with the technological tandem, it's not just about accomplishing more—it's about finding the right balance and doing it as naturally and sensibly as possible.

We do need to discuss the future of energy healing, or quantum healing, as it relates to the past, the present, and what's yet to come. First, let's cover some definitions, as that will help you as you go through the rest of the book.

DEFINING OUR KEY TERMS

When we say "technology," we're usually talking about contemporary devices, tech that is powered by electricity, powered by batteries, digital—everything from smartphones to computers, wearables to serious science machines such as MRI scanners, and those little wirelessly operated plugs that let you control the flow of electricity.

However, another definition of technology is "the application of scientific knowledge for practical purposes." This is an important distinction that reminds us that technology is not inherently good or bad; technology is neutral and it is how we, as humans, use technology that defines its purpose and intention. For example, the digital communications that allow instant human-to-human contact around the world can also pose problems, ranging from the perils of information overload to privacy concerns. Clearly, what we do with technology—how we approach it—can be vital in defining its direction in our lives.

Next, let's define the core concept of this book. By *quantum* energy, we mean energy—you can't escape it; it is all around you, it is within you, and it is within all the substances around you. The quanta of energy are within the smallest building blocks of human life—our cells. It's kind of abstract, but bear with me, because this is the foundation of how all the machinery of the universe works at the deepest level. Frankly, you can also define it as consciousness. While many don't yet understand this, it's indeed what we talk about when we say *quantum energy*. Everything derives from consciousness. Taken a step further, everything even is consciousness. Active consciousness (like all living beings), and "locked" or "waiting" consciousness. That's the fundamental truth the ancient and modern healers all knew about.

So what does this have to do with healing? That's simple. Quantum energy is the driving force behind quantum healing. It's based on the idea that by accessing and manipulating these tiny energy particles, we can impact our body and, in turn, our well-being. It's about the notion of the body as being energetic, not simply physical.

But what do imbalances or blockages in energy tell us about physical illness or emotional disturbance? And how might the body be healed through the balancing and rebalancing of its quantum energy? These are a few of the fundamental questions this book tries to answer.

The harnessing of quantum energy anchors us to the energy healers of long gone civilizations. They might not have known the term *quantum energy*, but they do appear to have understood that humans are healthier when their energy is in balance. For example, acupuncture has utilized different energy meridians in the body in order to resolve imbalances for thousands of years, and it is essentially based on energy. Likewise, Reiki (healing energy) and Ayurveda both involve the careful realignment of our energy flow for the sake of promoting health.

Now, though, we can measure these energies and their effects with modern electron microscopes and biosensors. These practices are coming back not only because they are, at their roots, foundational, but because they have not gotten old; instead, they have been honed for thousands of years to be perfect for today's technical age.

With that understanding, perhaps we can find our way with a foot in each camp—and get the best of both worlds.

Connecting the Past, Present, and Future of Healing

Holistic healing is not a thing of the past. Let me repeat that, because it's important: Holistic healing is *not* a thing of the past. Most of the medicinal practices I went over in Chapter 1 are still being used today, often in conjunction with modern medical technologies and pharmaceuticals. Traditional Chinese medicine, especially practices like acupuncture and exercises like Tai Chi, is very much alive and well.

These ancient therapies have returned to favor as complementary forms of treatment to modern medicine. Acupuncture is seen as a cure-all; so are advanced shamanic healing practices. Tai Chi and Qigong are embraced for stress relief, improved cardiovascular health, and joint mobility. These approaches believe that becoming healthier physically requires practices established for their own sake, both individually and in the social context of others. Their beneficial effects can have an impact on the broader community.

Massage therapy can benefit advanced cancer patients by improving pain and mood. Post-breast cancer treatment fatigue can be reduced by yoga. You can manage new cancer symptoms with regular practice of Tai Chi or Qigong. These are only some of the health scenarios that have demonstrated that these ways of tuning up your body can have actual benefits—not just the feel-good fuzziness that they are sometimes accused of.

Research into these issues continues to mount, becoming more robust, increasingly detailed, and more optimistic. Body, soul, mind: It's not a battle for supremacy; it's an undivided union in this reality. These ancient techniques deserve to be part of modern healthcare as well.

You don't have to visit an ashram to take part in an Ayurvedic lifestyle, either. Practitioners can be found easily throughout the world, and most still use the methodologies and philosophies prescribed hundreds, if not thousands, of years ago. Why wouldn't they? As they say, if it ain't broke, don't fix it.

Ayurveda's focus on maintaining health is just as wide-ranging as any doctor's, encompassing the mind, body, and spirit. And treating all three works very well indeed. Its preventative approach to diet, herbal remedies, yoga, and meditation still works wonders every day. Modern Ayurvedic practitioners often supplement their traditional methods with contemporary medical knowledge and clinical research to provide a comprehensive approach to well-being.

The same can be said for Indigenous medicine. Many native cultures still practice their ancient ways today because they have thousands of years of knowing what works and what doesn't.

In some cultures, traditional healing systems contribute to national identity and are integrated into national healthcare systems. For instance, clinicians in Thailand may prescribe nonallopathic remedies, including locally grown herbs, as part of a holistic approach to healing that encompasses the well-being of extended kinship groups and local communities. This integration means that historically rooted modalities can work alongside modern medical systems, fostering a vast number of treatment possibilities and therapeutic options.

One thing we can all agree on is that each of these ancient healing traditions emphasizes the bond between people, nature, and energy. Each has its own way of relating the natural elements to the functions of the human body, be it a focus on four elements like the Greeks, or five elements like TCM or Ayurveda. The commonality between ancient healing practices can also be seen in the theme of life forces being in or out of balance.

If we can connect the dots and find the common themes between a number of ancient healing practices, how can we also find the common thread that ties the past to the present and on to the future? That's what brings us back to energy. What we know now that our ancestors didn't is that the energy they were trying to tap in to is real and quantifiable.

Energy is the one thing that connects us across the generations, across the miles, across the millennia. And here, in the 21st century, we have the technology to understand it in a new way. That's one of the reasons why technology is not necessarily the enemy. We just need to use it to our advantage. Use it for good, not evil. Make the choice for the constructive and positive.

HEROES OF MODERN HOLISTIC HEALING

Holistic healing informed by traditional methods is happening globally with contemporary healers who claim remarkable results.

Mohan Sadashiv Joshi: Growing up in India, Joshi has used what he calls "Yogic Healing" to treat supposedly untreatable diseases for nearly 40 years. To improve an individual's state of wellness, Joshi asks participants to place one hand on their head and another on their back while he prays over them.

He says he has had success for "every kind of disease, from the common (migraine, insomnia) to the rare (Multiple mitochondrial dysfunctions syndrome (MMDS), a genetic disorder that is now considered to be a mostly incurable disease)." Joshi holds healing workshops both remotely and in person. He reminds participants that his "healing shakti" (divine power to heal) comes from God, not from himself.

Richard Gordon: Founder of a contemporary holistic healing technique known as Quantum-Touch, Gordon has a global appeal, as he promises to "transport you into the future of energy healing." Gordon developed this procedure in the 1980s and 1990s. His Quantum-Touch technique of energy healing is based on specific exercises involving breathing and body awareness that are meant to enhance the body's ability for self-healing.

Many of those who have received the treatment give a glowing account of the various applications of Quantum-Touch: "bone and structure alignment happens easily and quickly," "injuries from sports heal fast," "pain relief," "reduction of the signs and symptoms of chronic diseases," "reduction of pain after surgery," "healing of scars and burns," "relief from frozen shoulder," "weight release," and "emotional healing."

In medical practice, chiropractors, osteopaths, vets, surgeons, dentists, massage therapists, physical therapists, sports professionals, and athletic coaches have written to say that they had good success with Quantum-Touch. Sick animals have also benefited from Quantum-Touch as documented by Dr. Ronnie Turner, founder of the Chiropractic Association of Ireland, who noted that Quantum-Touch enabled him to "drive hips and bones back into place."

Barbara Brennan: One of the first pioneers of energy medicine and a leader in the field of energy healing, Brennan moved from a career as a NASA physicist to founding the Barbara Brennan School of Healing. She became a noted author in the field, publishing the New Age classics *Hands of*

Light: A Guide to Healing Through the Human Energy Field and *Light Emerging: The Journey of Personal Healing.*

These books detail her body-focused methodology, which is rooted in both hard science and spiritual insight. She illustrates her approach throughout her books, but one of her main ideas is that profound physical, emotional, and spiritual healing can be facilitated through an understanding of anatomy and the human energy field.

Eric Pearl: As an energy healer, Eric Pearl is perhaps most famous for his development of Reconnective Healing. This process is intended to reconnect the body's energy lines with the grid lines of the universe, "allowing any health and well-being issue to be resonantly absorbed and transcended."

According to his website, Eric suffered a series of extraordinary events in March 2000 that led him to discover his ability to reconnect others. Pearl claims to have healed others through the technique and published his book *The Reconnection: Heal Others, Heal Yourself.*

His manual describes the techniques of his type of energy healing, noting it "requires working with the frequencies of energy, light, and information that is easily accessible—that moves us beyond healing at a physical level ... to healing at all levels of our being." Pearl has taught his techniques via global seminars and workshops, training thousands of practitioners of energy healing worldwide.

Choa Kok Sui: Choa Kok Sui devised his signature form of pranic energy healing in the late 20th century. His books, including *Miracles Through Pranic Healing* and *Advanced Pranic Healing*, specify and systematize much of the practice. In his writings, Sui's version of energy healing synthesizes the ancient psychotherapeutic practices of the body-emotion system with current scientific understandings of the biological body. It adheres to the traditional notion that the body is largely self-repairing and that ailments stemming from the energies of the body-mind system (prana) can be treated with energy medicine.

According to Pranic Healing theory, the invasiveness of Western medicine disrupts the body's self-repairing system while energetic medicine repairs the body's energy field, so its self-repairing can occur more efficiently. The practice manipulates prana to facilitate the healing of ailments.

In his training of various disciples, Sui created a fully fleshed-out energy medicine practice that differentiates between the energy body and the physical body, even as it also suggests that they are essentially the same body. It includes practical teachings on energy cleansing, using the hands to read the energies of the body-energy and conscious energy systems, and delivering specific protocols for various ailments. The Pranic Healing practice can be found worldwide through its ranks of practitioners and its own global network of teaching facilities.

Donna Eden: Donna Eden is a renowned energy medicine teacher and author who has been teaching ways to tune in to and work with personal energies for over 30 years. Eden shares and instructs on "hands-on" techniques for self-care through her books *Energy Medicine* and *Energy Medicine for Women*.

Her approach blends the practices of traditional Chinese medicine, acupressure, and other related methodologies into a user-friendly system designed for balancing energies to maintain wellness. Her teachings aim to empower individuals to manage their own health and energy flow effectively.

Rosalyn Bruyere: Rosalyn Bruyere is an American energy healer and clairvoyant, and the author of *Wheels of Light: The Chakra System as a Blueprint for the Body, Energy, and Healing*. She is a leader in the healing and spiritual development movement and founded the Healing Light Center Church in California.

Bruyere's work with chakras focuses on channeling energy through the body for healing, providing a structured approach to understanding and utilizing the body's energy systems for health and spiritual development.

These healers, among many others, illustrate the diverse approaches to energy healing and the potential for achieving good health through a better understanding of the body's energy systems. By integrating ancient wisdom into contemporary methods, they offer practical techniques for improved wellness in today's world.

Roman Christian Hafner: Roman Christian Hafner has the ability to see and describe energy fields—a gift he was born with. He uses this ability as a mentalist, coach, and energy healer, and he has trained hundreds of other energy healers throughout Europe for more than 18 years. He regularly gives seminars and has been featured on various TV, radio, and online media channels in Switzerland, Germany, and Austria.

Since Roman has internalized the energetic principle and the frequencies of all creation levels, he can look into the molecular structure of any matter—even over distance. While Roman was born with the ability to see, isolate, and transform individual frequencies, it took him some time to truly hone this skill.

Cru von Holtzendorff-Fehling: Cru von Holtzendorff-Fehling was born with the ability to see energy fields and people's auras. As a coach, Alpha Chi teacher, and energy healer, Cru has coached and helped countless individual and business clients in Europe, the U.S., and Asia for about 20 years. The essence of Cru's work is to provide a space of unconditional love in which all reflection finds ground for growth and healing.

She helps her clients find clear, optimal solutions for their personal and spiritual growth. Her ability to read the most intricate energy systems and souls allows her to create abundant spaces for healing, filled with unconditional love and acceptance.

Johannes Koller: Johannes Koller is a clairvoyant energetic and trauma healer. He is president and founder of the Harmony Academy, which has several hundred active members. Johannes's work focuses on promoting a balanced and peaceful existence for all living beings, including humans, animals, and plants.

Johannes has also developed a unique trauma-healing method that goes deeper than traditional energy healers. His approach addresses all levels of the body, mind, and soul, which allows for genuine realization and the transformation of trapped energy into positive, freely accessible life energy.

We Are Frequency

Once you begin to understand that everything, including us, is made up of quantum energy, it's easy to realize that in order to truly be well, we must resonate at the optimal frequency for our health. Left alone to nature, our bodies will do that. We will harmonize with the natural frequencies around us and within us. And if those frequencies were to get scrambled or out of sorts, it's nature, that ancient medicine of medicines, that would heal us.

Our bodies are adept at self-regulation. In nature, our galvanic skin responses help maintain our core temperature within safe limits. Plant vibrations help regulate our body's electrical frequencies and biorhythms, and the color cycles of sunlight help maintain our circadian rhythms. These connections are not just poetic; they have scientific and bio-electrophysiological significance.

But as a modern society, we've gotten too far from nature for that to happen on its own. We no longer live in the forest, drink from the rivers, or turn to herbs to soothe our ailments. We live near high-voltage power lines. We cook our food in microwaves.

We allow doctors to send X-rays, ultrasonic waves, and magnetic frequencies through our tissues to diagnose our illnesses. We carry cellular devices in our pockets. Technology isn't inherently bad, but it is resetting and impacting our body's natural frequencies—and we just let it. Electronic use has become so ubiquitous that we don't stop to think about the effects of being so far removed from nature.

These technologies have undeniably brought benefits, particularly in medicine, communication, and daily convenience. However, they come at a cost. The myriad electronic devices and artificial electromagnetic fields that envelop us disrupt our body's natural frequencies. This interference is so pervasive that we seldom notice it anymore.

Consider the long-term exposure to electromagnetic fields (EMFs) from our gadgets.

These EMFs can disrupt the body's electrical messaging system, affecting sleep, hormone production, and cellular healing processes. The blue light from screens suppresses melatonin production, disrupting our sleep-wake cycles. Constant exposure to Wi-Fi signals contributes to chronic low-level stress over time.

Our immersion in an electronic lifestyle makes it difficult to appreciate what we've lost. We seldom pause to consider the cumulative impact of living in such an electrically saturated environment. The conveniences of modern life often blind us to the subtle but profound ways it transforms our bodies.

So what can we do to reclaim the harmonious vibrations conducive to health and well-being? The first step is awareness. By identifying disruptive sources and understanding their effects on our bodies, we can start making different choices.

One practical step is reconnecting with nature.

Spend more time outdoors, practice "earthing" by walking barefoot on natural ground, and reduce exposure to artificial EMFs. Practices like meditation, yoga, and Tai Chi can align our frequencies with those of the natural world. Exposure to natural light, limiting screen time, and creating device-free zones in our homes can also help.

Additionally, technology itself can provide solutions. EMF shields, anti-static mats, and biofeedback devices can mitigate the adverse effects of our electronic age. By using technology wisely and balancing it with our natural connection, we can navigate the benefits of modern advancements while countering their drawbacks.

In the next chapter, we will delve deeper into these strategies, exploring practical approaches to restore and maintain our natural frequencies. By combining ancient healing wisdom with modern technological advancements, we can find a path forward that honors our past, enriches our present, and safeguards our future. Let's explore these options and begin with some first steps in the next chapter.

REFERENCES

1. Brennan, Barbara. (1993). *Hands of Light: A Guide to Healing Through the Human Energy Field*. Bantam Books.
2. Bruyere, Rosalyn. (2000). *Wheels of Light: The Chakra System as a Model for Energy Healing*. Simon & Schuster.
3. Choa Kok Sui. (2009). *Miracles Through Pranic Healing*. Institute for Inner Studies Publishing Foundation, Inc.

4. Eden, D. (2008). *Energy Medicine*. Penguin Life.

5. Hippocrates. (2002). *Hippocratic Writings*. Penguin Classics.

6. Höhn, C., Hahn, M. A., Gruber, G., Pletzer, B., Cajochen, C., & Hoedlmoser, K. (2024). "Effects of evening smartphone use on sleep and declarative memory consolidation in male adolescents and young adults." *Brain Communications*, 6(3), Article fcae173. https://doi.org/10.1093/braincomms/fcae173.

7. Joshi, M. S. (2021). *Yogic Healing Techniques*. https://www.healmohan.org/.

8. National Ayurvedic Medical Association, The (NAMA). (n.d). "What is Ayurveda? The Science of Life." https://www.ayurvedanama.org/what-is-ayurveda.

9. National Cancer Institute. (2024, October 31). "Complementary and Alternative Medicine." https://www.cancer.gov/about-cancer/treatment/cam.

10. National Center for Complementary and Integrative Health (NCCIH). (2019). "Acupuncture: Effectiveness and Safety." https://www.nccih.nih.gov/health/acupuncture-in-depth.

11. Nunn, J. F. (2002). *Ancient Egyptian Medicine*. University of Oklahoma Press.

12. Pearl, Eric. (2007). *The Reconnection: Heal Others, Heal Yourself*. Hay House Inc.

13. Quantum-Touch Inc. (2021). "What is Quantum-Touch?" https://quantumtouch.com/en/about-us/what-is-quantum-touch.com.

14. World Health Organization (WHO). (2013). "WHO Traditional Medicine Strategy 2014–2023." https://www.who.int/publications/i/item/9789241506096.

3
What If We Had a Device?

"If you want to find the secrets of the universe, think in terms of energy, frequency, and vibration."
—Nikola Tesla

While some people question Nikola Tesla's financial and business decisions, no one can dispute his genius. From an alternating current (AC) system to the Tesla coil, Tesla's technological contributions were quite amazing. Tesla's inventions were frequently visionary; ahead of his time, they were sometimes even seen as science fiction dreams. The dream of wireless world power today seems strangely prophetic as new technologies have moved inexorably toward Tesla's ideas, and his proposal of harnessing natural planetary frequencies has become a recurring feature of new-wave cosmology.

The Serbian-American scientist and inventor spent much of his career working on machines that definitely fit the theme of this chapter: What if we had a device ...?

We concluded our last chapter by asking another question: What are we going to do about the fact that much of our modern technology is resetting and rearranging our internal energy waves? Of course, there's no one answer. Today, we live in a world of myriad electronic devices that, from cell phones to

Wi-Fi routers, microwave ovens to medical imaging equipment, produce an array of frequencies, all the while interacting with our biological systems. Many offer a great deal of upsides, but they similarly open a Pandora's box of new challenges to our system running by natural energy rhythms.

It's a big question, so let's use this time to explore some possibilities. We'll go with a little bit of science, a little bit of science fiction, and a little bit of blue-sky thinking to brainstorm about a device that could protect our bodies and our energy from the disruption of external waves.

What could such a device actually look like? A device we could actually wear or carry or put near us that would protect us from electromagnetic pollution while also optimizing our internal energetics would be ideal. The better the device, the more integrated with our lives it might be, accommodating our current modes of operation (smartphones, wearable tech, and the like) in order to account for our high level of addiction to these kinds of gadgets.

Such a device would need to build on current technology but go well beyond current capabilities. It could make use of exotic new materials with unusual kinds of conductive properties, incorporate new algorithms to identify and cancel intrusive frequencies, and rely on quantum principles to enhance beneficial energies.

Here's my stab at the device's emergent capabilities: renewable energy devices (daylight and others); fusion power cores (magnetohydrodynamic); fission power cores (nuclear); electric engines; various motors; internal combustion engines; kinetic energy devices (gyroscopic pendulums); charging hubs for phones, laptops, and so on; organ donations (healthy cell tissue); Wi-Fi signals; meteorological data; radar burst signals; telemedicine data; credit cards (contactless); TVs; hi-fi systems; laptops; PCs; iPads/tablets; music players.

That's just off the top of my head. Tesla had little to draw on except physics and his own imagination. He envisioned a different kind of world—pulsating with energy but spewing out less pollution—and he dreamt it into being. Why couldn't we do the same? That's the opening I'd like to explore.

Crafting such a device will be an innovative journey for sure, but with some help from the creative world of science fiction, where anything is possible, we can begin to assemble a future filled with devices that can not only support the utility of our energy but also extend to the care and protection of the earth.

DRAWING FROM POP CULTURE

If you're like me, you can instantly think of a device identified in a piece of pop culture that now either exists or is likely to exist in the next five to ten years. I tend to go straight to *Star Trek*—communicators seem like cell phones writ small, right? But I want to think of a device that can copy, transmit, and amplify information and frequencies as well.

Of course, the transporter beam might be an obvious choice. But how close are we, as a species, to having the physics and energy sources in place to actually decompose someone's molecules and reassemble them in a different place? As much as I love quantum energy, I'm not certain I'd jump at the chance to be a beta tester for a transporter beam.

Instead, let's look back even further, to Isaac Asimov, Ray Bradbury, Robert A. Heinlein, and Philip K. Dick—the great old masters of science fiction. They built us worlds of mind-bending machinery, artificial intelligence, and (almost) frictionless space travel. Although known universally for *2001: A Space Odyssey's* "too"-smart computer, HAL9000, Arthur C. Clarke also peppered his novels with a technology he called "matter organizers."

What's a matter organizer, you ask? According to Clarke, it was a device that could cause a computer-generated image to be constructed as a real object. A 3D printer, in other words. Clarke predicted the 3D printer 30 years before the first patent was filed for stereolithography.

The gist of my sci-fi ramblings is that if humans can dream it, humans can do it. We can look to the great thinkers that have come before, whether they are scientists like Tesla or wordsmiths like Clarke. The uncanny inventions, real or fictional, that dot the works of the previous centuries tell us that, yes, we can achieve the impossible.

DOES THE TECHNOLOGY EXIST?

So if our intention is to seek out or create a device that can copy, transport, and amplify information, and we want that device to also neutralize and harmonize potentially harmful frequencies, do we have the technology? (Brings to mind another sci-fi favorite, *The Six Million Dollar Man*. They had the technology to make him better, stronger, faster!)

What materials do you think would be best for a device like the one I'm describing? Would it be something large? Small? In between? How would it work?

Copying Information and Energy

A core feature of our dream device will be its ability to copy information and energy. Copies are already part of a host of technologies that partially realize this goal. Data can be copied and stored in digital storage devices, and energy harvesters capture and store background and available energy from the environment. Technologies such as quantum computing are potentially capable of more sophisticated forms of data handling and energy processing, which might even enable us to work with energy at the level of individual quanta.

Transporting Information and Energy

Another crucial function is the capability to transport information and energy. There are well-known macroscopic examples for information transport, such as the internet and wireless communication, where information is moved worldwide in a matter of milliseconds. For energy transport, there is now wireless energy transfer, from the inductive charging of various devices to inter-vehicle communication (IVC) between vehicles and more advanced wireless power transfer (WPT) projects for electric vehicles. Tesla's vision of "world wireless" (the establishment of a worldwide wireless energy infrastructure) is being revisited and refined in modern research.

Amplifying Information and Energy

Amplifying information and energy are two other areas where we've made significant progress. Signal boosters and repeaters are used to amplify communication signals so that data can travel long distances at improved quality. In the energy domain, there are several examples of technologies that amplify energy, such as Tesla coils and approaches based on resonant inductive coupling. These technologies might fit perfectly into the design of the device we envision.

Neutralizing Potentially Harmful Frequencies

The elimination of harmful frequencies is perhaps the most interesting and important feature of our dream device. The most effective materials and technologies serve as preventative protections against EMF radiation. One such technology is BioGeometry, utilized by Egyptologist and research scientist Dr. Ibrahim Karim.

BioGeometry involves specific shapes that can harmonize biological energy systems, reducing negative effects. Another natural material is shungite, a mineral with a unique crystal structure that absorbs and neutralizes EMF radiation. This could be our "magic" material.

Harmonizing Potentially Harmful Frequencies

Balancing frequencies to create a harmonious energy field is also possible. Devices that create a Schumann resonance (the natural frequency of the earth itself) can "space charge" and harmonize human energy fields within the earth's electromagnetic waves. Such devices might find application in our dream device to maintain energy harmonization.

So there you have it. The problems exist, the skill exists, and the magic material exists. Now it's just a matter of time.

Imagining the Device

Considering these technological advancements, we are closer than ever before to creating a device that meets our specifications. The key point is to conceptualize how these technologies can be integrated. Metals alone might be semiconductive but not fully conductive; however, shungite could integrate with

BioGeometry and quantum computing to generate a multi-functional, relatively small device.

Imagine a device the size of a standard smartphone, embedded with a layer of shungite for EMF protection, BioGeometry shapes to harmonize energy flow, and quantum computing to process and magnify energy and information. This device could copy, transport, amplify, neutralize, and harmonize harmful frequencies.

As you ponder this thought experiment, consider which materials and technologies you might use. How would you design it?

Real-World Examples

To illustrate our capability, let's look at some real-world examples:

Li-Fi Technology: Scientists have invented light waves technology, known as Light Fidelity (Li-Fi), to transmit data similar to Wi-Fi. Li-Fi has the potential to replace Wi-Fi and help reduce exposure to radiofrequency radiations. This technology is currently being tested for various applications, showcasing human ingenuity in inventing and improving existing technologies.

EMF Shielding: Electromagnetic field shielding, in the form of fabrics and paint, is used to fend off fine-line and microwave radiation. EMF shielding products can be added to furniture, fabrics, and personal devices, demonstrating that modern technology can coexist with us by adapting our environment.

Wearable Health Monitors: Devices like Fitbit, Apple Watch, and other health monitors record health data such as steps taken, heart rate, and sleep patterns. This data is relayed back to the wearer in real time, helping us better understand our bodies and live healthier lives.

Do We Have the Capability?

Aside from our ability to dream up the wildest inventions and devices, humans are uniquely equipped to build them. We have the knowledge, physiology, and capability to draft plans, gather materials, and use tools to complete their creations. To me, it's absolutely incredible—the machines and technologies that we've created as a species are mind-boggling.

Nevertheless, the evolution of humankind hasn't moved as quickly as the evolution of our technology. We aren't physiologically designed to handle the bombardment of electromagnetic energy fields and frequencies put off by the creations we've invented and integrated into our daily lives.

That's why our "dream" device is so critical. Since we can't expect everyone to give up their microwaves, cell phones, and medical diagnostic tools, we have to be intentional in our desire to build something that we can use to counteract the impacts of the frequencies emitted by those devices.

What if I told you that the device, the one that meets all our parameters, already exists and that I had a hand in creating it? Now what if I told you that we actually have several devices that meet the specifications, and some are small enough to carry with you everywhere? Well, it's true, and I'm so excited to tell you about them. Let's go to the next chapter, and I'll fill you in on all the details.

(And by the way, I wasn't pulling your leg about thinking about possibilities or making sketches. I want you to dream big and use your problem-solving skills; you could come up with the next big thing in quantum energy devices. The world needs more of them, trust me.)

References

1. Bahr, F. (2016). "Li-Fi: Data transmission via LED." *International Journal of Computing and Digital Systems*, 5(4), 297–305.
2. Baraniuk, C. (2018, October 11). "How light could help superfast mobile reach even further." BBC News. https://www.bbc.com/news/business-45811959.
3. Hull, C. W. (1984). "Apparatus for production of three-dimensional objects by stereolithography." (U.S. Patent No. 4575330A). U.S. Patent and Trademark Office. https://patents.google.com/patent/US4575330A/en.
4. Karim, I. (2009). *Back to a Future for Mankind: BioGeometry*. BioGeometry Consulting Ltd.
5. Kurotchenko, S. P., Subbotina, T. I., Tuktamyshev, I. I., Tuktamyshev, I. Sh., Khadartsev, A. A., & Yashin, A. A. (2003). Shielding effect of mineral schungite during electromagnetic irradiation of rats. *Bulletin of experimental biology and medicine*, 136(5), 458–459.
6. Lewis, T. (2023). "Has the 3D printing revolution finally arrived?" *The Guardian*. https://www.theguardian.com/technology/2023/mar/12/3d-printing-the-new-technology-comes-into-its-own.
7. Norman, D. A. (1993). *The Design of Everyday Things*. Doubleday.
8. Simões, F., Pfaff, R., & Freudenreich, H. (2011). "Observation of Schumann Resonances in the Earth's Ionosphere." *NASA Technical Reports Server*, 20120000051. https://ntrs.nasa.gov/citations/20120000051.
9. Tesla, N. (1900, June). "The Problem of Increasing Human Energy." *Century Illustrated Magazine*. https://teslauniverse.com/nikola-tesla/articles/problem-increasing-human-energy.
10. Yanofsky, N. S., & Mannucci, M. A. (2008). Quantum Computing for Computer Scientists. Cambridge University Press. https://www.cambridge.org/core/books/quantum-computing-for-computer-scientists/8AEA723BEE5CC9F5C03FDD4BA850C711#fndtn-contents.

4
Science and Implications

"Equipped with his five senses, man explores the universe around him and calls the adventure Science."
—Edwin Hubble

Now that you know we have devices that fulfill all our requirements for quantum energy disbursement and protection, I'm sure you're curious about how they work. These devices represent a remarkable convergence of cutting-edge technology and ancient healing principles. They're designed to enhance your well-being in a world saturated with disruptive frequencies. As we delve into the science and implications of these devices, you'll discover how they harness quantum energy to create a harmonious environment for you and your loved ones.

In this chapter, we'll explore the reality of these devices, backed by rigorous scientific studies and certifications that validate their effectiveness. We'll uncover the intricate mechanisms that allow them to copy, transport, amplify, neutralize, and harmonize energy. From understanding the materials used in their construction to examining their impact at the cellular level, you'll gain comprehensive insight into how these devices can transform your health and environment.

Let's dive right in and talk about the fascinating science and technology behind these revolutionary quantum energy devices.

THE REALITY OF THE DEVICES

The reality of the devices is that they are cutting-edge quantum energy technology meant to help you live a healthier, more harmonious life. Made of the finest materials, premium metals, and advanced fabrics, all have been tested for their conductive and protective properties, particularly in quantum energy. This ensures that every material and component is chosen for its efficiency in interacting with and channeling quantum energy.

All these devices come in different forms to fit the various needs of daily life. They are in the form of blocs, which come in several different sizes to allow targeted applications. The frequency capsules and cards provide easy-to-use energy protection wherever you go. The pet collars ensure that your pet is balanced with well-harmonized energies too.

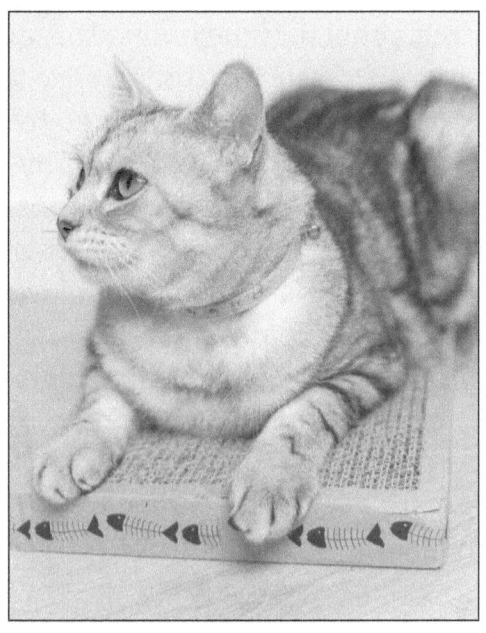

Specialized pet collars can help cats and dogs feel the effects of quantum energy too.

There are also water bottles that, when filled, will infuse your drink with quantum energy and supportive frequencies (for example, of important vitamins, minerals, and organic plant extracts), and they turn regular water into structured high-energy water. All these products are developed for a specific purpose and infused with the ability to harmonize, or precisely resonate, with specific frequencies to ensure maximum benefits for you, your family, your pets, and your environment.

And if you're feeling a little skeptical of these devices, you're not alone. Many people don't understand the potential of quantum energy, nor how we can capture it for personal use within our devices.

This skepticism is exactly the reason why so many laboratory studies have been performed to verify the effectiveness of these quantum energy devices. These studies aren't just hypothetical; they prove, empirically, how these devices protect us from the damage of the many external frequencies to which we are constantly exposed. The quantum energy devices have been subjected to all kinds of studies and different testing methods to confirm their protective and restorative abilities: from petri-dish studies in the lab to real-world user trials, all carefully controlled and scientifically sound, with practical applications.

THE SCIENCE BEHIND THE RESULTS

Studies and certifications are one way we can tell the world that these quantum energy devices are real, effective, and capable. I'm proud to say that in addition to numerous independent studies, our devices have been studied and certified by two of the world's leading authorities on biosystem and bio-informational analysis as well as EMF research and testing: the BESA Institute in Austria and the IGEF Institute in Spain and Ireland. Furthermore, the products are LifeSpan certified, and the capsules won the Dragonfly Health Innovation Award in 2024.

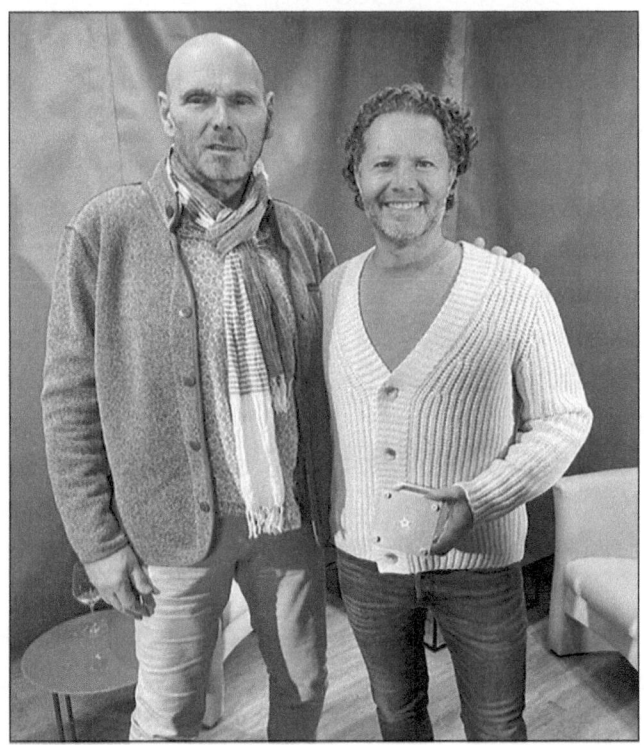

With the head of the BESA Institute, Wolfgang Albrecht.

These certifications prove that the science works—our quantum energy devices function as intended and have measurable positive effects on health. IGEF studies on our H.E.A.L. Capsule show that the protective effect of the device even increases with the duration of use, as it does with many of our devices. That means the longer you use them, the more profound and positive the effects will be.

This is consistent with reports of chronic, cumulative improvement among our users as they attest to incremental improvements to their health and well-being over months of use.

Another interesting study using our devices was a structured water analysis conducted by the Emoto Institute in Japan. Structured water is believed to promote higher energy levels; improve sleep, memory, and concentration; detoxify the body; and support better digestion and a stronger immune system.

When the Emoto Institute studied the effects of our devices on water, they saw a significant, positive change in distilled water within only three minutes with the weakest bloc. Within ten minutes, our water bottle had optimized the water it held, making it structured for maximum benefits and informing it with the frequency data of important vitamins and minerals. That's powerful stuff!

These findings, based on our own scientific knowledge and experience as practitioners, offer very practical and tangible benefits to users of these quantum energy devices. That's why the structured water analysis makes sense. Improved water is one of the best medicines there is—on a molecular weight level, our bodies are over 99 percent water. Fascinating, right?

IMPROVING BLOOD FLOW

One of the most remarkable things about our quantum energy devices is their effect on humans at the very cellular level—specifically, the blood. This flow must always be steady, which means that each red blood cell should have space between it and others, plus a little wiggle room. This allows each cell to come and go at a steady pace, avoiding crushing or congestion and ensuring everything to do with the blood can happen efficiently. This means things like waste removal, oxygenation, phagocytosis, and other immune functions can take place without any cells crashing into the cells next door.

Have you ever been caught in a crowded room where there is no sense of flow? You just want to get to the exit, but there's no space to breathe, let alone move. It's chaotic, and it makes you feel stressed and tense. That's what happens to our blood cells when they're exposed to the chaotic frequencies of things like microwaves, Wi-Fi, cellular signals, and other EMF emissions.

When blood is stressed, the critical coagulation cascade is activated early and part of the clot sticks to the walls of the blood vessel. Over time, these clots build up and stick together, potentially leading to hypertension, heart attack, stroke, or other serious issues.

Here's the cool thing: Our quantum energy devices can not only reverse that chaos but also actually help improve your blood flow to optimal levels. Several independent placebo-controlled dark-field microscopy studies (conducted in the U.S. and Austria) support these findings. Baseline blood samples from each showed moderately organized and functional, good but not great, cells. Following the sample's exposure to Wi-Fi, the cells became clumped and compressed with limited motion and excessive space around the cells—evidence of stress.

After treating these blood samples with quantum technology, they looked quite different. Our quantum devices stimulated the bodies of all test participants to entirely reverse this cellular chaos, putting blood back into its ideal state of flow. The cells regained their ideal structure and showed no further signs of stagnation in their movement. Furthermore, within the bloodstream, the cells were no longer clumped or compressed. Additionally, white blood cell activity and motility increased, which is important for the immune system. It's absolutely incredible to see these results on a cellular level.

In addition, our devices have the advantage of not only counteracting the negative effects of EMFs. They also actually promote regenerative processes and self-regulation that boost all your body systems toward their optimal function. This means that our quantum energy devices can vastly improve our overall well-being in a way that cannot be realized with the often symptom-centric treatments of conventional medicine. People often tell us that after using our products they have more energy, they sleep better, and they've become sharper mentally and physically. Even pets get perkier and calmer.

MORE ATP PRODUCTION

Another study result that shows significant promise is the increase in adenosine triphosphate (ATP) production. When different types of human cells were subjected to quantum energy, including healthy fibroblast cells, ATP levels increased by 20–29 percent for a few hours before returning back to baseline. This effect was consistent across different types of cells and experiment setups.

Why does ATP matter? If you think back to your high school biology class, you'll remember that ATP is the energy your body's cells need to do work. With a 20 percent boost, your cells could speed up regeneration, repair, and recovery. Temporary ATP boosts could also improve endurance and reduce downtime between physical activities, which maximizes workout sessions. Increased ATP production in brain cells could improve cognition and might even be able to protect neurons during the process of aging.

You get the idea—ATP is pretty important. Although this is just a preliminary study, it shows enormous potential for the benefits of quantum energy on the human body.

Enhanced Cell Recovery

I'm going to share one more big result with you, because I think it's tremendously important. It's about cell recovery. Researchers wanted to see if a quantum energy field could help skin cells heal faster. They used human dermal fibroblasts (skin cells that play a role in wound repair) and created a small "scratch" in a layer of these cells in a lab dish.

The cells were divided into two groups: one exposed to the quantum energy field and one not. Over several days, researchers took pictures of the scratch to measure how quickly it healed in each group. To ensure fair results, the study used a double-blind design, meaning neither the researchers nor those analyzing the results knew which group was treated.

The cells exposed to the quantum energy field healed much faster than the cells that were not. The treated cells showed improvements ranging from 45.8 percent to 100 percent faster compared to the untreated cells. And it wasn't just a one-off result: The quantum-energy-exposed cells consistently healed more quickly across multiple experiments conducted over a year.

If these findings can be confirmed in further studies, including in humans, the technology could have significant benefits for health and well-being. Faster recovery from injuries, such as cuts, scrapes, or surgical wounds, might reduce discomfort and the risk of infection. It could also help treat chronic wounds, particularly those that heal slowly due to conditions like diabetes or poor circulation. It could enhance skin regeneration, offering potential advantages for cosmetic procedures or treatments for skin conditions. Faster healing could lead to reduced medical costs by shortening hospital stays, decreasing the need for dressings or wound care products, and minimizing complications.

The possibilities are pretty astounding, when you think about it.

THE PROOF IS VERIFIABLE (AND UNDENIABLE)

Our quantum devices have been the subject of no fewer than 59 studies, the majority of which were placebo-controlled, and new studies are always underway. We're also always looking for ways to improve and boost the effectiveness of the devices because helping people reach their peak quantum wellness is our calling and top priority. EMF emissions are not going away any time soon. It's imperative that we continue finding new ways to utilize quantum healing energy.

Here are some of the most notable results of the studies conducted:

1. The devices reduce stress, improve sleep quality, and increase cognitive function.

2. Participants using our devices reported fewer and weaker symptoms of electromagnetic hypersensitivity, including headaches, fatigue, and dizziness.

3. The devices support cellular repair mechanisms, helping people recover faster from the effects of physical overexertion.

4. The devices elevate the naturally occurring abundance of certain oxytocin genes associated with bonding and empathy, and this increase lasts for several hours after usage.

5. Use of these devices and quantum energy showed an increase in cellular ATP production.

The question remains: How will you use these devices to improve your well-being? While this section of the book has been a brief overview of the technology and science of the devices, I invite you to continue reading. In the next few chapters, we're going to explore all the practical applications of the devices for you, your family, your home, and your environment. The true potential of quantum energy is in your everyday life.

References

1. BESA Institute. (n.d.). BESA Institute. https://besaguetesiegel.com/ueber-uns/fachverband/.
2. BESA Institute. (n.d.). "Independent Studies on Quantum Healing Devices." BESA Institute. https://besaguetesiegel.com/ueber-uns/fachverband/.
3. Emoto, M. (2013). *The Hidden Messages in Water*. Atria Books.
4. IGEF Institute. (n.d.). International Association for Electrosmog Research IGEF Ltd. http://www.elektrosmog.com.
5. IGEF Institute. (n.d.). International Association for Electrosmog Research IGEF Ltd. (2020). *Expert Opinion for the biophysical investigation of the Leela Quantum und H.E.A.L. capsule.* https://leelaq.com/wp-content/uploads/2020/10/12.10.2020-Gutachten-Leela-Quantum-and-H.E.A.L-1.pdf.
6. Mitchell, I. (2024). "Impact of quantum energy on cellular ATP production." International Quantum Technology and Frequency Medicine Association. https://ifqtf.org/atp-study-impact-of-quantum-charging-on-human-cellular-energy-production/.
7. National Institute of Environmental Health Sciences. (n.d.). "Electric & Magnetic Fields." National Institute of Environmental Health Sciences https://www.niehs.nih.gov/health/topics/agents/emf.

8. Rubik, B. (2022). "Leela Quantum Bloc shows protective effects on the blood upon human exposure to short-term Wi-Fi." International Quantum Technology and Frequency Medicine Association. https://ifqtf.org/wp-content/uploads/2024/04/Rubik_Leela_Quantum_Bloc_Protects_the_Blood_Jan_2022_REV_2_POSTED.pdf.

9. Sheaff, R. J. (2024). "Investigation of Leela Quantum Bloc Technology and its effects on wound healing." International Quantum Technology and Frequency Medicine Association. https://ifqtf.org/wp-content/uploads/2024/04/Leela-Quantum-Bloc-Technology_Wound-Healing.pdf.

10. World Health Organization. (n.d.). "Electromagnetic fields." World Health Organization. https://www.who.int/india/health-topics/electromagnetic-fields.

Section 2:
The Practical
Use of
Technology

5
Humans

"No matter the circumstances, joy is always the best medicine for any mental or emotional pain. Find joy in anything and you will reset your moment for a more fulfilled next moment in your life."
—Cru von Holtzendorff-Fehling

What's the use of having incredible quantum healing technology if you don't incorporate it into all your activities? Whether you're on the go or spending time at home, quantum healing can be a vital part of your day with some amazing practical applications.

Quantum healing devices are completely noninvasive and totally safe to use. Certain conventional treatments require medication with possible side effects or surgical procedures, but quantum healing is a completely natural, gentle way to help facilitate the healing process. This makes them perfect complementary therapies to act alongside conventional medical treatments you may be undergoing at the same time.

Imagine drinking some structured water in the morning to ensure optimal hydration and motivation. Imagine a night of restful and rejuvenated sleep because you blocked the energies that were disturbing your slumber, allowing you to have more productive days. Imagine tempering minor strains or subtle imbalances of immune function, or enhancing the mind's clarity and emotional stability by building up its "quantum energy."

All of this and more is at your fingertips with our technology. Let's explore some ways quantum healing can work for you, no matter what you're up to.

STRUCTURING YOUR WATER

Structured water, sometimes called hexagonal water, is water that has had its molecular arrangement altered to boost its natural properties. The better hydrated your cells are, the better your overall health. Quantum devices have the power to structure your water, which may help you reap the benefits of improved cellular function and increased sustained hydration. Structured water keeps you hydrated, and hydrated cells are better at absorbing nutrients and removing waste. Structuring your water with a quantum device also supports better energy and more attuned frequencies.

When water molecules line up in their ideal hexagonal structure, they pass more easily and readily through cell membranes, providing more thorough hydration at the cellular level. That's staying hydrated in the proper sense of the word. Structured water doesn't just hydrate; it enhances your cells so they operate at optimal cellular efficiency and vitality.

Finally, the molecular order of hexagonal water is also thought to carry high levels of body energy and influence your body's frequency for perfect alignment. The improved structure is believed to be more conducive to energy flow within your body, which results in more stamina and vitality.

Incorporating structured water into your daily life is easy to do and potentially life-changing. Drinking structured water daily will provide sustained improvements in hydration, nutrient absorption, elimination of toxins, and increased energy. This one small change can shift how you feel and function, paving the way to a healthier path and a more balanced life, and creating a canvas for you to stand taller in the world.

IMPROVING YOUR SLEEP QUALITY

Protect yourself from negative energy and get the best night's sleep when you have quantum healing technology in your sleep space. It can help you feel calmer, more relaxed, and in tune with your best sleep frequencies.

There's little to no need for unnatural sleep aids like medications when you have access to quantum frequency medicine, possibly in combination with some proven natural substances like chelated magnesium, glycine, and so on. Aside from using devices to support a calm, sleep-conducive atmosphere, you can also use quantum technology to charge your favorite bedding with the frequencies that promote your best sleep. Quantum frequencies can be a game-changer for partners and families—if one person's snoring is a disruptor for the whole household, think of the peace and calm that will come with improved sleep energies. As everyone knows, when you get a good night's sleep, you're better equipped to take on whatever the next day brings.

Quality sleep is also an important part of maintaining overall physical health. A good night of sleep improves your cognitive well-being, your immune system response, and your skin—giving you extra energy and that elusive youthful glow. With quantum healing, you not only sleep better but also get better benefits from your sleep as your body's natural processes improve to provide more energy, a better mood, and a more alert mind.

If left untreated, anxiety or mental preoccupations, even mild confusion, can be the result of ongoing stress, continual exposure to digital screens, overexercise or undernutrition, as well as exposure to toxins and a wide range of environmental stressors. These subtle energy imbalances can all contribute to poor sleep quality. Quantum healing is a holistic approach to a full night's rest because it helps rebalance these subtle energy imbalances with a healthy, natural approach to restful sleep.

PROMOTING HEALING

Quantum healing is called that for a reason. Things happen that throw us out of our most healthy state of balance; that's part of living the human life. Quantum healing devices are an exceptional tool for what happens. Use them to change the healing frequency of your bumps and bruises. Perhaps the best feature of quantum healing is that it speeds your recovery by putting your body in sync with its own natural healing frequencies, so you bounce back quicker.

Quantum healing devices help reduce everyday aches and pains. Whether you have slight discomforts such as aching legs or back from overexertion, fatigued feet, headaches, muscle pain, or superficial sprains and strains, quantum healing can help ease discomfort and assist in the quickest possible recovery. By resetting the body's healing frequencies, quantum healing supports the body's natural healing mechanism. It allows you to feel better, quicker.

Besides addressing your physical problems, quantum healing devices may also boost the effects of the medications and supplements you have taken. Charged with beneficial frequencies by your quantum healing device, they help you to get as much benefit from your treatments as possible. Using quantum healing to address your health challenges from the inside out is a much more comprehensive healing approach than anything traditional Western medicine can provide.

Some quantum devices can even help you heal others through the power of intentions. Simply place their photo or something belonging to them in or near your healing device and watch them begin to improve, no matter where you or they are in the world. That's the incredible thing about quantum healing; energy frequencies can travel great distances to serve a purpose where needed.

Quantum healing isn't just for when you're feeling out of sorts. Using these devices in your daily life will maintain your body's energy and keep you well. It's an overall well-being enhancement. You can connect the dots from mind-body medicine to psychoneuroimmunology to wellness and self-care. Through the principle of quantum entanglement, your energy self-balances, which means you can enjoy better mental focus and emotional equanimity. Optimal energy balancing will also improve your physical health.

MANIFESTING ENERGIES AND INTENTIONS

It's easier to manifest your goals when you've got the power of quantum healing and quantum energy on your side. It's all about using your quantum device to tap into the frequencies that will help you achieve what you've set out to do or be.

Whether you've set goals for health or wealth, vitality, or detoxification, or you just want to boost your positive energies, there's a device to help you manage frequencies for whatever you want to manifest in your life. Once you discover the incredible power of manifesting your intentions through quantum energy, you will begin to wonder how you ever achieved anything without your quantum devices.

PROTECTING YOURSELF FROM EMFs AND 5G

I've saved the "best" for last—at least, the everyday application that I wish everyone in the world would get on board with. We spend our lives bombarded by frequencies, and if we don't protect ourselves from the harmful ones and purposely surround ourselves with the beneficial ones, we could all be permanently damaging our bodies' cellular structure and causing real, irreparable damage.

Electromagnetic fields, or EMFs, are everywhere, and while many are naturally occurring phenomena, we, as a human society, have introduced many more unnatural EMFs. Power lines, electronic devices, electric lights, Wi-Fi signals, and cellular radiation like 3G, 4G, and 5G, not to mention appliances like microwaves, assault our bodies with frequencies not attuned to the earth or our cells.

Some people suffer from a condition known as electromagnetic hypersensitivity (EHS), and those with the syndrome claim that they can feel EMFs radiating through them and disrupting their bodies' natural cellular order. Add in medical technology like X-rays, and it's a wonder we aren't all a mess of dysregulated cells just trying to survive.

That's where quantum healing devices come into play. They break down and break through the electrosmog of EMFs and promote the frequencies your body needs to rest, relax, and heal from such intense stress on a cellular level. With the EMF and 5G protection of quantum healing technology, you can feel more powerful and energetic and be bold, spontaneous, and vibrant, even in a world that aims to keep you fatigued and flat.

TESTING NEW APPLICATIONS

If you're thinking that all these practical applications are amazing, you're right. But maybe you're also thinking, "What else can quantum healing do for me?" We're asking that question too, and we're constantly trying to find new, exciting ways to use quantum healing devices and technologies.

For now, quantum healing is largely an uncharted territory filled with possibilities. Researchers and practitioners have countless questions about how quantum devices might address a whole host of issues related to physical and mental well-being, from healing skin to aiding the immune system. This, in turn, can interact with the environment to ameliorate disease in other ways, including through various toxins and electromagnetic fields (EMFs) that abound in modern environments.

The best thing we can do is use the quantum technology we have now as we continue to develop a more advanced and more powerful quantum technology of the future.

REFERENCES

1. Emoto, M. (2004). *The Hidden Messages in Water*. Atria Books.
2. Havas, M. (2008). "Electromagnetic hypersensitivity: Biological effects of dirty electricity with emphasis on diabetes and multiple sclerosis." *Electromagnetic Biology and Medicine*, 25(4), 259–268. https://doi.org/10.1080/15368370601044192.
3. Karim, I. (2007). *Back to a Future for Mankind: BioGeometry*. BioGeometry Consulting Ltd.

4. Mild, K. H., Repacholi, M., van Deventer, E., & Ravazzani, P. (2006). "Electromagnetic hypersensitivity: proceedings, International Workshop on Electromagnetic Field Hypersensitivity, Prague, Czech Republic, October 25–27, 2004." World Health Organization (WHO) Press.

5. Momoli, F., Siemiatycki, J., McBride, M. L., Parent, M.-É, Richardson, L., Bedard, D., Platt, R., Vrijheid, M., Cardis, E., & Krewski, D. (2017). "Probabilistic Multiple-Bias Modeling Applied to the Canadian Data From the Interphone Study of Mobile Phone Use and Risk of Glioma, Meningioma, Acoustic Neuroma, and Parotid Gland Tumors." *American Journal of Epidemiology*, 186(7), 885–893. https://doi.org/10.1093/aje/kwx157.

6. Murphy, M., Donovan, S., & Taylor, E. (1997). *The Physical and Psychological Effects of Meditation: A Review of Contemporary Research With a Comprehensive Bibliography*. Institute of Noetic Sciences.

7. Nilsson, M., & Hardell, L. (2023). "Case Report: Both Parents and their Three Children Developed Symptoms of the Microwave Syndrome while on Holiday near a 5G Tower." *Annals of Clinical and Medical Case Reports* 12(1), 1–7. https://acmcasereport.org/wp-content/uploads/2023/12/ACMCR-v12-2046-1.pdf.

8. Peterson, C. T., Denniston, K., & Chopra, D. (2017). "Therapeutic Uses of *Triphala* in Ayurvedic Medicine." *Journal of Alternative and Complementary Medicine*, 23(8), 607–614. https://doi.org/10.1089/acm.2017.0083.

9. Rubik, B. (2002). "The biofield hypothesis: Its biophysical basis and role in medicine." *Journal of Alternative and Complementary Medicine*, 8(6), 703–717. https://doi.org/10.1089/10755530260511711.

10. Schiffman, S. S., & Nagle, H. T. (1992). "Effect of environmental pollutants on taste and smell." *Otolaryngology—Head and Neck Surgery*, 106(6), 693–700. https://doi.org/10.1177/019459989210600613.

11. Schoen, A. M. (2001). *Veterinary Acupuncture: Ancient Art to Modern Medicine*. Mosby.

12. World Health Organization. (2010, May 17). "Interphone study reports on mobile phone use and brain cancer risk." (Press release No. 200). https://www.iarc.who.int/wp-content/uploads/2018/07/pr200_E.pdf.

6
Plants

"Plants know how to make food and medicine from light and water. They know how to keep the Earth safe and protect their children. Plants teach us that good energy is found in reciprocity, in giving and receiving generously, and in honoring the relationships that sustain life."
—Robin Wall Kimmerer

Quantum healing technology isn't just for humans; it's also beneficial for plants. For those of us who garden or find joy in keeping houseplants, we already know how special it is to nurture life. When our favorite flower blooms or we harvest food to nourish ourselves and our loved ones, it brings a rush of satisfaction and gratitude for the generous nature of beautiful beings.

The silent assistance of plants shows how to use light and water resources to create life-sustaining foods, how to nurture the earth's surface back into balance, and how to cultivate trustworthy relationships so all species can thrive in the co-creative web of mutual help. When we apply quantum healing to gardening, we improve our crops, practice stewardship, and respect the give-and-take caring partnership that underlies cooperative ecology.

In this chapter, we will explore several practical applications of quantum healing as it applies to plants and discuss how this cutting-edge technology can help you to create a lush space filled with beautiful, healthy plants. Whether you are an avid gardener or a devoted caretaker of houseplants, you will learn how quantum healing can help you give back to plants and make this life more colorful, green, full, and bountiful for all.

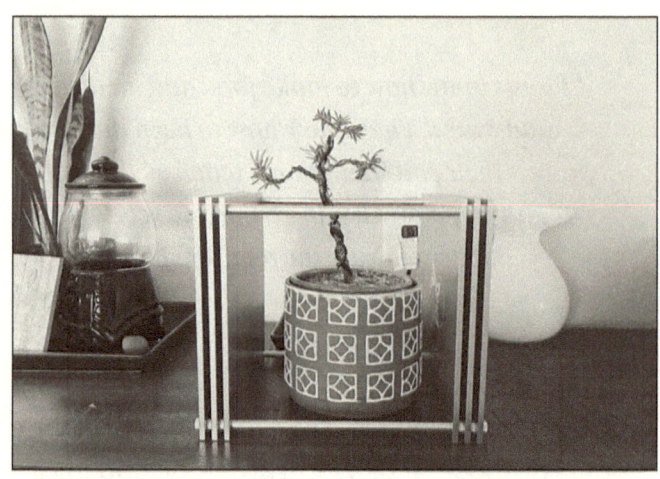

An Infinity Bloc from Leela Quantum Tech can help mitigate the effects of electromagnetic fields (EMFs) on houseplants.

PREVENTING PLANT DAMAGE

Just as our human cells can be damaged by electrosmog, so, too, can our plants. Think about the food you might grow in your vegetable garden or orchard; do you want to consume food that comes from a plant bombarded by EMF energy?

If you don't mind me saying so, it's counterproductive for us to protect ourselves from electrosmog and then eat a tomato that's been altered by the very thing we want to shield ourselves from. That's why it's critical to use quantum healing devices to protect our plants. We also need to protect the plants we keep in our living spaces; not only do they deserve, like all living things, to live their healthiest lives, but also we don't want anything we enjoy enough to keep nearby to be the recipient of harmful energies.

This is why quantum healing devices are indispensable when it comes to guarding our food and plants from harmful energy. When carefully positioned as bio-shields, they serve as both a kind of electronic immune system and a means to protect plants from destructive electrosmog. The result sustains the integrity of the plants and their ability to produce healthy, unadulterated food.

Ultimately, keeping our plants safe from electrosmog is just the logical extension of our wider efforts to create a cleaner, healthier space for ourselves. Using quantum healing technology in your gardening routines as well as in your plant care can offer your plants the best of both worlds, improving their lives, the food they produce, and the spaces in which they grace us with their presence.

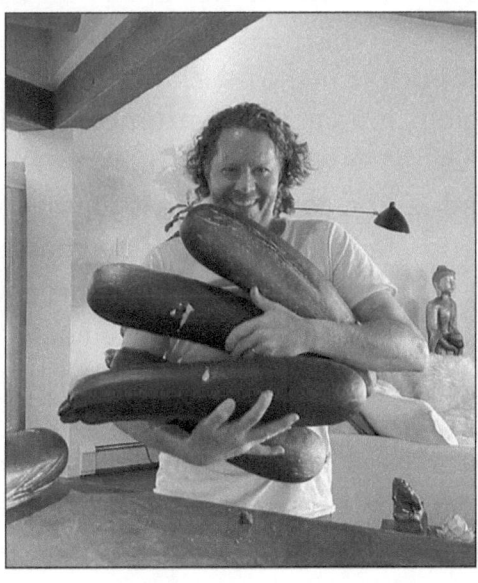

We placed an Infinity Bloc from Leela Quantum Tech in our garden and since then our vegetables have flourished.

Supporting Photosynthesis

Let's go back to the idea of structured water and how it helps our human cells function on a more optimal level. It can do the same thing for your plants by promoting the effectiveness of plant cells on a molecular scale.

Regular access to structured water may improve the effectiveness of photosynthesis. Keeping your plants hydrated with structured water means they can potentially excite more molecular movement and more efficient photosynthesis. The more they can photosynthesize, the larger they can grow, and the more they can produce.

The structured water will synergize with the quantum healing devices and the whole will then be greater than the sum of its parts.

Extending the Life of Cut Stems

As we've discussed, one of the benchmark qualities of quantum healing technology is its ability to promote healing and boost vitality. If you've cut flowers from your garden or received a gift from someone, you can extend the life of your lovelies by using structured water in the vase to supercharge their energy.

If you don't have ready access to structured water, another useful technique is to charge the vase itself before using it. You can do this by putting the vase inside a quantum healing bloc until its energy is properly charged. The charged vase will then maintain the structural integrity and well-being of the flowers by infusing them with this positive energy so that the flowers remain healthy and vibrant for as long as possible.

If you have cut stems that you want to root into new plants, quantum healing can also protect the stems while they're vulnerable and promote faster root growth so you can plant your new plants in much less time.

Placing the cut stems near a quantum healing device puts out structured frequencies that will help prevent environmental stressors or disease. The structured water used in watering the cuttings will also support the stems' cell functions much more than common tap water, giving your new plant the best possible chance to thrive right from the start.

ENERGIZING SEEDS BEFORE PLANTING

Want to grow bigger, stronger, and healthier plants? Start by energizing your seeds. If there's one thing that gardeners love to do, it's experiment, so try this: Grab four or six of your favorite vegetable seeds, and charge half of them with quantum healing frequencies. Then plant all of them.

Water the charged seeds with structured water and the non-charged seeds with regular water. Watch what happens when the plants grow. The energized seedlings given structured water will not even seem like the same plant species as your non-energized, non-structured-water seedlings. The power of quantum healing and plant production is mind-blowing, especially when you start from seed.

ENSURING BALANCE IN YOUR GARDEN

Like all living things, plants each have their own frequency— every blade of grass, every tree, every flower, and every vine. If you've got a garden, then you have a ton of competing frequencies. When plants are grown too closely together, the frequency of one may compete with that of another, causing them to get out of balance. This can result in stunted growth.

The plants may not be healthy, and their productive yield can be impaired. Each plant emits a certain frequency, and each of these needs to be balanced with every other plant.

If you've ever been to the symphony, you know the cacophony of every-player-for-themselves warm-ups until the concertmaster brings them all together in one glorious tuning note before beginning the performance. That's what your garden feels like without quantum energy to harmonize it. A quantum healing device can help you bring your garden into balance, ensuring that every plant can grow and thrive without drowning out the frequency of another.

A quantum healing device emits frequencies of energy that "speak" to all of the plants in your environment via their frequency "voice." The plants' fields of energy respond and follow these resonating frequencies. By keeping them in a state of coherence, the plants become integrated and function together as a whole. When the plants' fields of energy are lined up, they don't interfere with one another and they more easily grow and thrive together.

EXPLORING OTHER PRACTICAL USES

Plants are amazingly responsive beings. Have you ever watched a parched, wilted plant seemingly spring back to life after a good watering? It may seem miraculous, but it's just a testament to the resilience of cellular-based life and how well it survives when given what it needs.

One practical use with widespread potential application is in large-scale farming where seed germination rates are of crucial importance. By treating seeds with quantum healing devices just before planting, farmers can pre-enhance germination rates by a measurable amount. Energized seeds may lead to healthier seedlings.

This use extends to structured water as well. When plants are watered with structured water from quantum healing devices, the roots absorb and use more nutrients from the soil, resulting in stronger, healthier plants with increased growth rates and stronger resistance to diseases and pests.

There is still another step in the commercial farming process that can take advantage of quantum healing before entering the market: post-harvest technology. If the food has only a few days of shelf life, quantum options can really become a viable and important alternative. Quantum healing frequencies can treat the fruits and vegetables so their cell vitality lasts longer, even after they have been harvested. The concept is simple: The longer the shelf life, the less food gets wasted, the more profitable it is for the farmer, and the fresher it stays for the consumer.

There are even more promising opportunities for quantum healing technology in space agriculture. If human beings are going to colonize other planets in the near future, quantum healing apparatuses could help create a nurturing space environment for plant growth, possibly onboard a space station or even on an alien planet. If quantum healing can enable plants to thrive in a non-earth environment, it will be instrumental in ensuring sustainable food sources for our space explorers.

Looking even further down the line, quantum healing technology could be employed on larger scales to prevent famine and ensure the availability of food worldwide. Through the use of quantum devices, crops in areas with poor soil quality, drought, or other poor environmental conditions could be improved and made more resilient and productive. This would also help buffer famine in areas where populations are vulnerable and help ensure an adequate global food supply.

And that's just the beginning! The applications of quantum healing for plants are endless. From optimizing seed germination to making space agriculture a reality (and everything in between), the applications for quantum healing technology are limitless as well as exciting. And with the ever-increasing number of novel applications that we may discover in the future, the possibilities for developing more sustainable agriculture, as well as turning our backyards into beautiful, lush, and nutrient-rich gardens, are endless.

REFERENCES

1. Ayesha, S., Abideen, Z., Haider, G., Zulfiqar, F., El-Keblawy, A., Rasheed, A., Siddique, K. H. M., Burhan Khan, M., & Radicetti, E. (2023). "Enhancing sustainable plant production and food security: Understanding the mechanisms and impacts of electromagnetic fields." *Plant Stress*, 9(100198). https://doi.org/10.1016/j.stress.2023.100198.
2. Creath, K., & Schwartz, G. E. (2004). "Measuring effects of music, noise, and healing energy using a seed germination bioassay." *Journal of Alternative and Complementary Medicine*, 10(1), 113–122. https://doi.org/10.1089/107555304322849039.
3. Emoto, M. (2004). *The Hidden Messages in Water*. Atria Books.
4. Kimmerer, R. W. (2013). *Braiding Sweetgrass: Indigenous Wisdom, Scientific Knowledge, and the Teachings of Plants*. Milkweed Editions.
5. Pierce, M. (2021, November 23). "NASA Research Launches a New Generation of Indoor Farming." National Aeronautics and Space Administration (NASA). https://www.nasa.gov/technology/tech-transfer-spinoffs/nasa-research-launches-a-new-generation-of-indoor-farming/.
6. Rein, G. (2019, November 29–30). "Effect of Structured Water on Plant Growth and Metabolism." [Conference presentation]. Bionutrient Food Association 2017 Soil & Nutrition Conference, Stockbridge, MA, United States. https://www.youtube.com/watch?v=V676M4YuT1A

7. Tolle, E. (2008). *A New Earth: Awakening to Your Life's Purpose*. Penguin Group.

8. Vian, A., Davies, E., Gendraud, M., & Bonnet, P. (2016). "Plant Responses to High Frequency Electromagnetic Fields." *BioMed research international*, 2016, 1830262. https://doi.org/10.1155/2016/1830262.

7
Animals

*"Until one has loved an animal, a part of
one's soul remains unawakened."*
—Anatole France

Animal people come in all varieties, from the "pets are people, and this is my fur baby" type to the "exotics or bust" type to the dyed-in-the-wool generational livestock farmer. One thing all these types of animal lovers have in common is that they only want what's best for their animal companions, whether they are a pampered pooch, a parrot or python, or a prizewinning pig. Quantum energy healing can assist with that.

Animals will also benefit from the diverse, practical, everyday uses of quantum energy healing. For pet owners and even livestock caretakers, this technology becomes an additional tool in their arsenal to create a harmonious, calming, and productive environment: to ease pain, discomfort, or improve the life of their beloved pets or livestock.

CREATING A POSITIVE ENVIRONMENT

Animals experience and emit frequencies very differently than humans. They are extremely sensitive to any changes in frequency and attuned to EMFs in ways that humans simply aren't built for. For example, if you place a human in an EMF field and then charge the EMF, they might not even notice; on the other hand, a cat or dog, because of their sensitivity, will literally seek shelter if the electromagnetic environment starts to climb.

Any small change can dramatically affect their stress levels and ability to function. Luckily, this also means that you can create a carefully charged environment that supports their health and well-being using the power of quantum healing devices. In a study of the effects of quantum energy on dogs, a bioenergetic systems analysis (BESA) showed a huge shift from stressful energy to balanced energy.

You can create safe spaces for each animal in your life by energizing their pet beds, cages, terrariums, stalls, and barns with frequencies that best suit their needs.

Consider how this can be applied across various settings:

Pet Beds and Cages: You can make your pet's bed or cage a sanctuary of peace and well-being using the energy and essence of crystals. This can be especially beneficial to pets like dogs in carriers or birds in cages, who are confined to small spaces for a good part of their days. By calming the energy of the space, you lower your pet's anxiety, making it easier for them to sleep, relax, and be at ease.

Terrariums and Aquariums: Birds, reptiles, and amphibians are extremely vulnerable to environmental changes. Placing a quantum healing device near a terrarium or aquarium could stabilize the microenvironment so that the life within will remain healthy and stress-free.

Stalls and Barns: Placing energizing quantum healing frequencies in the stalls and barns of larger animals such as horses, cattle, and other livestock can create an overall positive environment, making them feel more content. It will also lead to an improved sense of well-being in your animals.

Outdoor Areas: Devices can also be placed in outdoor settings for optimal health and behavior of animals that spend time outside in paddocks or grazing pastures.

If you take these proactive steps, you can be confident that you're creating a receptive environment, using the power of quantum healing to configure a place that enables your cat, dog, steer, or even llama to thrive.

RELEASING EMOTIONAL BLOCKAGES

Animals have feelings too, and just like humans, they don't always know how to express them. Because they can't verbalize their emotions, pets can often get "emotionally blocked." They can feel confused by changes in their routine or environment, sad about losing a human or other animal companion, and unsettled or even angry when things feel out of their control.

These blockages can often manifest as changes in their behavior, eating patterns, and general demeanor. For example, a pet whose personality suddenly changes—becoming withdrawn or downright aggressive—might have emotional issues underpinning the behavioral changes. When quantum healing energy is at the right frequency, your animal(s) will start to feel more like themselves again.

Regular quantum healing sessions will help your pet clear emotional blockages. Simply place your pet near a quantum healing device so they can absorb the frequencies. Even something as simple as giving them structured water rather than tap water can begin to free up their negative energy and boost their emotions. It can be helpful to integrate quantum healing practices into your pet's daily regimen, especially during times of stress, such as when moving to a new home or welcoming a new family member.

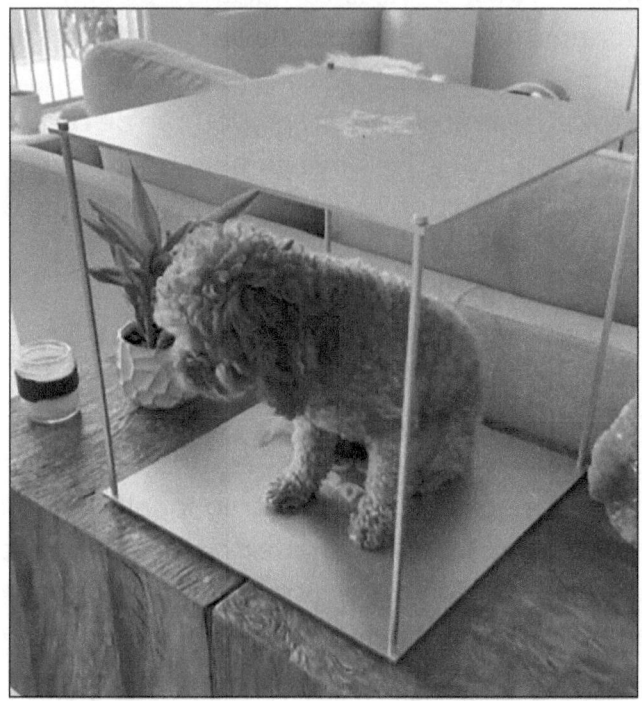

Cats, small dogs, and other animals can fit entirely inside a Grand Bloc from Leela Quantum Tech.

EASING PAIN AND DISCOMFORT

Like with humans, quantum healing technology applied to animals can help with energy levels, mobility, and sleep quality. This requires you to be attuned to their frequencies and know when something feels "off." Fortunately, those who are close to their animal companions, be they house pets or livestock, tend to harmonize with their frequencies, whether intentionally or not. This is why we humans who love our animals seem to know almost immediately when something isn't right with them.

Older animals can experience many health problems as they age, similar to how humans suffer as they grow older. Osteoarthritis is a common issue, in which stiff and swollen joints lead to pain and a significant decrease in mobility. Quantum healing technology can be a great help in these cases. With a device that emits healing frequencies, you can target painful areas and stiffening joints to bring about pain relief. Regular sessions with a quantum healing device can keep your mature pets more active and reduce their need for pain medications.

As animals grow older, digestive issues also become more prevalent. Gastrointestinal problems like gastritis and colitis can cause significant discomfort, loss of appetite, and low energy levels. You can assist them with this discomfort by using healing energies and intentions through your quantum devices. Combining structured water with quantum healing sessions can also aid in digestive processes, making it easier for pets to absorb nutrients and feel more comfortable.

Even if your pet shows no outward signs of suffering, regular quantum healing sessions can bring many benefits through preventive maintenance. Maintaining youthful energy frequencies can stop many age-related issues before they even have a chance to begin.

STIMULATING SELF-HEALING ABILITIES

Animals are incredibly resilient creatures. We've all heard stories of livestock who survived natural disasters against all odds or pets who've been adopted from terribly abusive situations and begun to thrive. Quantum energy can help stimulate and sustain your animals' natural self-healing abilities.

Biologically speaking, the frequency of the healing vibes alleviates more cellular damage, thus reducing the time needed to heal and keep the animal stronger and more mobile during the time of recovery. While the injury might take more time to heal, the quantum healing technology is a great complementary method to use. This way, the animal is helped not only physically with its injury but also mentally and emotionally through the healing process.

It's not just physical trauma that animals suffer from, it's also emotional trauma. These traumas leave energetic, emotional, and psychological scars in the animal's body and being. Quantum healing aids emotional recovery by energetically balancing the high- and low-frequency energy fields of the heart and the head. As the animals improve, they exhibit a drop in their heart rate, blood pressure, ventilation rate, and skin temperature, indicators of better health that reflect happiness.

If your pet ever gets injured or needs a medical procedure like surgery, you can set them up for a successful recovery with quantum healing technology that boosts their natural ability to heal themselves. With the right frequencies and intentions, your animal companion will be back on their feet in no time and feeling better than ever.

CALMING ANXIETY IN PETS AND LIVESTOCK

Living with anxiety long-term takes its toll, and finding relief can make an extraordinary difference—for humans and animals. Some animals feel and act nervous in new situations and around new people; some don't care for thunderstorms or other loud noises; and separation anxiety in house pets is a very real concern. The power of quantum healing energy to alleviate anxiety cannot be understated. Just as it helps you feel calmer and less stressed, it can do the same for animals.

Quantum healing using sound frequencies can calm pets or livestock by balancing and harmonizing the animal's energy field, leading them to a state of peace and calm. Placing a quantum healing device in areas of your pet's living space where they spend more time is especially helpful.

Structured water also helps with pet anxiety. Using structured water can connect you to your pet on a more emotional level and contribute to more positive cellular function. Even simple changes, like replacing your pet's regular tap water with structured water, can help them feel more balanced and less anxious.

Regular quantum healing sessions can also significantly aid anxiety management for nervous animals. For instance, if your dog gets anxious about thunderstorms, schedule a quantum healing session during the storm to help them stay calm. For livestock, quantum healing can be beneficial during stressful times, such as transportation to a veterinarian's office.

PROTECTING ANIMALS IN NEW WAYS

We're constantly thinking about new ways we can protect our animal companions and help them live happier, healthier lives. When we care for our pets, keep them safe from the same electrosmog that threatens our own well-being, and potentially extend their lifespan by easing their negative energies and ailments, we reap the rewards of being able to love and care for them longer. It's a win-win situation.

Many pet owners and livestock farmers report that their animals are much less anxious and more relaxed after regular exposure to quantum healing frequencies. Among the many testimonials, a favorite comes from a pet owner who said her dog showed less extreme separation anxiety—no longer destroying the doorjamb—and seemed much happier overall.

Another individual reported that livestock became calmer and more compliant during transportation once quantum healing devices were installed in barns and transport vehicles.

Here are some practical tips to maximize the effectiveness of quantum healing on animals:

Pay Attention to Stress Triggers: Watch your pets and livestock to identify what triggers their anxiety. The more you know, the better you can apply quantum healing techniques.

Create a Quantum Calming Space: Use quantum healing devices in an area designated as a calming space for your animals, such as a room for pets and a specific area in the barn for livestock.

Regular Healing Sessions: Incorporate regular quantum healing sessions into your animals' routine, especially during known stressful situations like thunderstorms, fireworks, or transport.

Provide Structured Water: Replace tap water with structured water to help your animals relax and feel happier overall.

Wearable Devices: Make use of wearable quantum healing devices on your pets to provide them with continuous support.

Incorporating quantum healing into your animal care routine fosters a well-rounded approach to your furry friends' health and well-being. By considering the whole animal—physically, emotionally, and energetically—you can achieve overall balance. Set aside a few minutes each day for face-to-face chats with your pets to assess their behavior and well-being, and place quantum healing devices strategically in your home and on their bodies.

Daily Energy Boosts: Create structured water and healing frequencies for your pets to consume daily.

Relaxation Areas: Designate areas in your home for your pets to decompress.

Continued Use: Take portable quantum healing devices with you during travel to maintain your animals' protection and balance.

Moving Forward with Quantum Healing: Outside of healing injuries, quantum healing technology promises to expand creature comforts and build a better world for all.

If this section of the book has you curious to learn more about quantum healing and wondering how you can use your knowledge to help others, then you need to move to the next chapter! I'll explain how you can become a certified quantum healer and be part of the next wave of quantum technologies.

REFERENCES

1. Dong, V. N. K., Tantisuwat, L., Setthawong, P., Tharasanit, T., Sutayatram, S., & Kijtawornrat, A. (2022). "The Preliminary Chronic Effects of Electromagnetic Radiation from Mobile Phones on Heart Rate Variability, Cardiac Function, Blood Profiles, and Semen Quality in Healthy Dogs." *Veterinary Sciences*, 9(5), 201. https://doi.org/10.3390/vetsci9050201.

2. International Association for Quantum Technology & Frequency Medicine (IFQTF). (n.d.). "Exploring the Effects of Quantum Upgrade on Blood Health and Energy Balance in Pets." https://ifqtf.org/exploring-the-effects-of-quantum-upgrade-on-blood-health-and-energy-balance-in-pets/

3. Lindinger, M. I. (2021). "Structured water: effects on animals." *Journal of Animal Science*, 99(5), skab063. https://doi.org/10.1093/jas/skab063

4. National Research Council (U.S.) Committee on Assessment of the Possible Health Effects of Ground Wave Emergency Network (GWEN). (1993). "Assessment of the Possible Health Effects of Ground Wave Emergency Network." National Academies Press (U.S.). https://www.ncbi.nlm.nih.gov/books/NBK208988/.

Section 3:
An Action Plan

8
Awakening Your Healing Potential

"Health is a state of complete harmony of the body, mind, and spirit. When one is free from physical disabilities and mental distractions, the gates of the soul open."
—B. K. S. Iyengar

Have you ever had a moment when you just knew that someone was hurting? Do you sometimes feel an unexplained compulsion to reach out to a stranger? Have you ever felt a sudden, inexplicable urge to comfort a friend before they've even said a word? These are all subtle signals of your innate healing abilities. The first step to becoming a certified quantum healer is recognizing these gifts: the intuition, empathy, and communion with others that are your healing abilities.

Intuition is knowing what someone else is feeling or experiencing without them saying anything about it. Often, we describe this in terms of inner voices or gut feelings, for example, "There's something about this person that bothers me," or "I have an inkling that this person won't help you with your problem."

Empathy is the capacity to feel what another person is feeling and live in their story as they continue to tell it. With a developed level of empathy, you can feel others' pain and understand their experiences on a whole-body emotional and sensory level. These qualities enable you to tune in to the other person to guide you in knowing how to help and provide the appropriate energy interventions needed for healing.

I remember a particular instance early in my journey when empathy profoundly shaped my approach to quantum healing. A close friend was going through a rough patch, struggling with chronic pain that left her exhausted and despondent. As I sat with her, listening to her recount her daily struggles, I found myself tuning in to her pain on a deeply empathetic level.

I could feel the heaviness in my own body, a mirror of what she was experiencing. This connection allowed me to intuitively understand where she needed the most support and how to channel healing energy effectively. By aligning my energy with hers and focusing on the areas of intense discomfort, I was able to help alleviate some of her pain, offering her a much-needed sense of relief and hope. This experience taught me the incredible power of empathy in healing, reinforcing the importance of truly connecting with others to provide meaningful support.

PRACTICES TO AWAKEN HEALING POTENTIAL

You don't need much to get started with healing—in fact, let's dive in right now! Tune in to the energy fields that weave through and around you. With these simple yet powerful practices, you can begin to unlock and cultivate your healing potential.

Contemplative Practices

Seeing Stars: Try to visualize the flowing energy lines of another person extending out from them, like radiant stars. See them glowing like emanations of loving, wise, and compassionate energy. This practice helps you tune in to the subtle energy fields of others, fostering a deeper sense of empathy and connection, and enhancing your ability to channel positive energy toward healing.

Contemplation of Universality: Visualize "drops" oozing down from the feet of another, and mentally recite "dripping, dripping, dripping." Continue this practice until the distinction between yourself and others, and the flow of energy and goodness from others to yourself, all fade away. This exercise promotes a sense of oneness and interconnectedness, breaking down barriers between self and others and allowing for a free flow of healing energy that can benefit both the giver and the receiver.

Meditation: Meditation can help you become more aware of your energetic aura and of the energetic auras of others. By practicing and deepening your meditation, the skillful awareness of scattered and overflowing energy used in grounding becomes more integrated and powerful. One of the most common forms of meditation, being mindful about your present-moment experience and the feelings in your body, can help develop your awareness of your energy field and your capacity to sense and transmit energy to others.

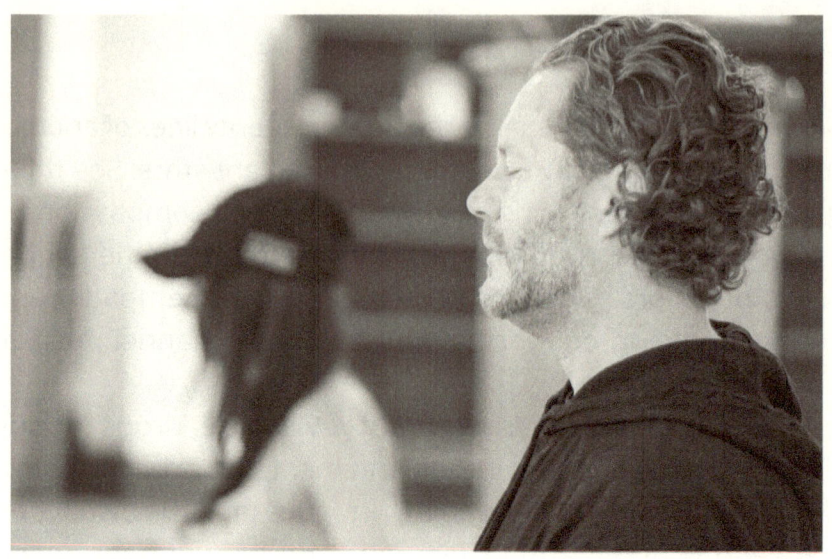

Leading a meditation session at the Dragonfly LIVE conference in 2023.

Mindfulness: Pay attention to your thoughts, feelings, and sensations moment to moment without judging yourself or the experience. This creates an awareness that enables an individual to become more sensitive to the energetic shifts that are occurring inside them and around them.

Other Contemplative Practices: Journaling, nature time, and creative pursuits can also increase energy sensitivity. Journaling helps you reflect on your experiences, notice patterns in your intuitive intelligence, and gain insights and emotional intelligence. Time in nature grounds you and helps you feel connected to the earth's primordial energies. Creative pursuits, such as painting, dancing, and making music, can organically direct your energies in positive ways.

Developing Consistency in Practice

Now that you have a variety of contemplative practices to choose from, the next step is to develop consistency. To get started, you'll want to incorporate these practices into your daily life to better open and fine-tune your healing skills. Begin with short sessions and gradually increase the length of time you can sustain your awareness. The main goal is to create a habit of attunement to your energy field and maintain levels of expanded awareness.

Increased sensitivity to subtle energy fields can be enhanced still further by a conscious practice of various exercises. There are, for example, the movement-based arts of Qigong and Tai Chi. These and other specific energy healing practices used to require traveling the world to find. They've gained popularity over the years, however, and it's very possible you can find an instructor in one of these ancient traditions near you.

In these disciplines, the very slow, deliberate, softly engineered movements of the body, often combined with purposeful breathing, controlled intention, and a clear-headed awareness of the senses and your own presence, can help develop your ability to feel more deeply into your own energy field. This practice can help you connect with layered or multi-dimensional aspects of yourself and engage more deeply with the "fifth" elemental force of nature, which is utilized in the practices of energy healers or movement practitioners.

There are no rules for this because there is no one right way to do it. However, it is helpful to engage with experienced healers or guides as mentors, if possible. They can watch your progress, give you feedback, help identify potential issues with your work, and help you make the most of the techniques.

Embracing Lifelong Learning

In order to become a certified quantum healer, you need to embark on a lifelong learning journey. The quantum healing field is constantly evolving and adding new insights, methods, and tools. Keep yourself curious; stay informed of new insights, methods, and tools; do not limit yourself to just one source but study with different masters; and remember that every experience can be a learning experience.

By identifying this essential healing aspect of yourself and incorporating these recommended practices, you can awaken and develop your skills, setting the stage for an even deeper journey into quantum healing.

My own journey began over a decade ago, and I still find myself learning new things every day. The beauty of quantum healing is that it's an endless exploration, where each new discovery opens doors to even greater understanding and capability. Embrace this journey with an open heart and a curious mind, and you'll find the path of a quantum healer is as rewarding as it is enlightening.

DEEPENING YOUR SPIRITUAL CONNECTION

Quantum healing requires a heartfelt connection with your spiritual self, since your ability to connect and focus healing energy comes from your soul. Since God is characterized as an energy field, an intimate relationship with the divine means that you can become a better transmission line for energy. Living from that center changes you and makes you more spiritually whole because you are more closely connected to it. There are many different ways of doing this, so use whichever path from among them suits you.

Intention Setting and Visualization

Intention setting and imagining future scenarios in which the body has healed are corollaries to quantum healing—using the mind to heal the body. It is a form of meditation in which thoughts are aligned to create desired outcomes. When we focus our mind, visualize what we want, and imagine our body healed, we are then able to harness energy in that direction.

What do you intentionally do to maintain, heal, or enhance wellness? It could be setting intentions (for example, you want to clear up your eczema and feel energized and bursting with vibrant energy). The very act of setting that intention channels energy and works subtly to move energy in the body to help you realize that goal.

You can visualize the body creating its own healing, or energy whizzing through your system, or you, at your perfect health. You can improve the link between the mind and body to promote your physical and emotional well-being. There is evidence to show that visualization can have physical outcomes such as pain reduction or better immune function.

Breathwork

Breathwork is a group of practices that uses slow, steady breaths, and sometimes holding the breath, to move and shift energetic patterns within the body. The goal is to forge a path to the nervous system, oxygenate the body, and promote relaxation and healing.

Controlled Breathing: Deep breathing, diaphragmatic breathing, and alternate nostril breathing calms the mind and body. Calming the mind and body reduces stress, lowers blood pressure, and enhances health. Focusing on one's breath creates awareness of the present moment, which enhances the ability to be at peace with one's self.

Pranayama: Pranayama is the practice in yogic systems by which the breath is controlled to influence the flow of *prana*, or life energy, in the body. Certain pranayama techniques, such as *Kapalabhati* (skull-shining breath) and *Bhastrika* (bellows breath), energize the body, shift energy blockages, and clear the mind. Regular practice of pranayama can increase vitality and reduce the effects of stress.

Holotropic Breathwork: Created by Stanislav and Christina Grof, holotropic breathwork is a practice that involves rapid, deep breathing through the nose to induce altered states of consciousness. This can lead to emotional release, increased spiritual insights, and profound healing. Participants report positive, characteristic experiences, including what one might call a general feeling of flourishing.

These rituals together form the foundation upon which quantum healing functions. They focus on balancing the body's energy fields so that they are aligned in the same pattern as when health is ailing due to various factors such as lack of attention to the body's signals, inadequate connection with the soul/psyche, poor diet, and so on. They also cover breathing, yogic practices, the power of intent and visualization, meditation, relaxation, and lifestyle techniques, among others. If they can be incorporated into daily life, they will bring about quantum healing.

Nature Immersion

There's perhaps no greater way to heighten the spiritual aspect of your life than by spending as much time as possible outdoors. Many people report that simply sitting in nature—a sunlit meadow, a wood, a riverside, the simplicity of a stone cairn surrounded by vibrant blooms—quiets their mind and helps them absorb natural energy from the earth in mini-meditative moments. It's easy to immerse yourself in nature:

- **Go Barefoot:** Ground yourself by walking barefoot on grass or soil.
- **Reduce Stress:** Nature quiets the mind, an ideal state for spiritual insight and healing.
- **Increase Awareness:** Being in nature invites you to be more present, attentive, and aware of the subtle energy fields and the interconnectedness of life.

Energy Work

Energy work such as Reiki is a direct way of connecting with an energy field. Have you ever seen Reiki in action? Reiki practitioners put their hands on the body and channel energy from the universal field to create balance in themselves and their clients. Energy work helps you to:

- **Increase Your Sensitivity:** The more you practice, the more sensitive you'll become to energy flows, and the more easily you'll notice disruptions and areas where energy needs to be restored.
- **Unblock the Channels:** Energy work is based on the idea that a blockage in your energy field is the root of disease, so healing it improves your health by restoring the natural sense of well-being.
- **Unleash Intentions:** Grounding universal energy sparks your therapeutic intent, expanding and strengthening it so your precious efforts really count.

Guided Visualizations

In guided visualizations, one creates images and visualizations and then focuses mind and mental energy to reconnect with the energy matrix and channel healing energy into patients or others. Advantages of guided visualization are as follows:

- **Focus and Clarity:** Visualization helps you to concentrate and clarify your healing intentions.
- **Emotional Healing:** Visualization can release negative emotions and promote emotional healing.
- **Sharpened Intuition:** Practicing on a regular basis helps develop your intuition so as to make better choices and be more responsive in the healing process.

Holistic Lifestyle

When you engage in a holistic way with "self" and adopt physical, emotional, and spiritual practices, you help establish a deeper and more meaningful spiritual relationship. This can be achieved through various methods:

- **Healthy Diet:** Eating a balanced, nutritious diet supports physical health and enhances energy levels.
- **Wearing Modest and Proper-Fitting Clothing:** Wear garments that allow air to circulate, avoiding tight-fitting or contrived styles. Wear loose-fitting underwear, socks, and shoes. Wear a cap or hat with holes to facilitate flow.
- **Physical Activity and Movement:** Do moderate amounts of exercise daily. If you engage in a yogic or Tai Chi-style exercise, practice it several times a day. Keep the chi flowing—don't let it stagnate.

- **Emotional Well-Being:** Journaling or therapy are good practices for keeping the auric field aglow and pleasant, containing the good energy.

With practice, you can learn to adopt some or even all of these methods in order to trigger the kind of spiritual engagement and quantum healing that will enable you to better tap into and direct energy for yourself as well as others.

Learning from Ancient Wisdom

Exploring ancient spiritual and healing traditions can inform and deepen your understanding of quantum healing in surprising ways. After all, they generally share a similar way of viewing the energy of the universe, the interconnectedness of all life, and the power of healing that exists not only within but also outside of ourselves, in the natural world. Here are some of the ancient practices and how they can contribute to quantum healing.

The tradition I've studied most is traditional Chinese medicine (TCM). Its profound understanding of energy flow, meridians, and balance has significantly influenced my approach to quantum healing. By integrating TCM principles with modern quantum techniques, I've been able to enhance my healing practice, bridging ancient wisdom with contemporary insights.

Ayurveda (India)

Ayurveda and quantum healing concur that good health is represented by a harmonious balance of bodily energies and systems. By blending the ancient Ayurvedic system with quantum healing, the complete human experience can enable people to reach new levels of health that serve as a buffer against disorders while healing the roots of disease for lasting well-being.

Quantum healing, like Ayurveda, is based on the concept that a state of corrected balance within one's energy fields allows for optimum health and well-being. Both of these systems believe that health is not just the negation of disease. Health means balance among one's body's systems of energy. Quantum healing also relies on using the idea of quantum vibrational energy fields throughout the body to achieve the correct kind of balance or coherence. Quantum healing supports the view that the healthy body is a balanced system of energy coupled with a system of information that generates health benefits.

In both Ayurveda and quantum healing, we have the use of a limited element—Ayurveda's three doshas and quantum healing's two vibrational energy fields (intuition and empathy). Through these, we can untangle imbalances, clinically diagnose and treat disturbances of the body, and establish correspondence between the physical and nonphysical realms in curing complex ailments. Both systems highlight the all-encompassing indivisibility of body, mind, and spirit; disturbances and healings of the body relate to the human condition, and balance among the three is essential for healthy life.

Ayurveda's use of color, herbs, and dietary interventions can all be correlated with quantum healing's techniques of energy color therapy, use of phytotherapeutic agents, and general holistic practice aimed at the maintenance of energy balance.

Traditional Chinese Medicine (TCM) (China)

TCM and quantum healing are similar in principle because they both embrace a holistic and energetic understanding of health as dynamic balance and harmony within biofield energy systems. These systems, when merged together, can boost the body's ability to heal itself by treating the source of the problem in ways that promote long-term vitality.

Perhaps the most obvious similarity, and the one most enticing from a scientific perspective, is the fact that TCM envisions the body as a vast energy system in which health is maintained by keeping energy flowing in the most optimal ways. In quantum healing, it is widely agreed that everything has energy or energy fields, and illnesses exist because energy flow and balance are disrupted, while health arises when physiological parameters and energy systems can resonate with one another in coherent, harmonic ways.

The concept of energy pathways that underpins quantum healing is similar to the meridian system of TCM. Just as acupuncture uses needles or lasers on specific points along the meridians to regulate the flow of chi, the goal of quantum healing is to direct energy fields to the optimal configuration used by healthy, vital cells and tissues.

The manipulation of energy forms seeks to replicate the body's natural processes working at optimal levels. Both acupuncture and quantum healing aim to correct these dysfunctions at energetic, or subvisible, levels to restore and enhance well-being. TCM practiced in the West acknowledges this holistic view of the body, mind, and spirit as a means to bring balance and health to the natural systems within and between us, the opposite of the reductionist workings of Western medicine.

TCM and quantum healing both promote prophylaxis and disease prevention as well as the maintenance of health through natural and noninvasive means. Using acupuncture, Tai Chi, and herbal medicine for treating or preventing illness in TCM resonates with practices within quantum healing based on energy balancing, meditation, and addressing illness with natural remedies that tap into the body's innate healing capacities.

Shamanism (Global Indigenous Cultures)

Both shamanic and quantum-based approaches to healing recognize that health is a state of well-being that involves an integrated and harmonious energy flow in the organism. Illness, by comparison, is a sign of dysfunction due to energy blockages that may stem from spiritual, emotional, or physical causes.

Quantum healing is based on the same principle as shamanism, that the universe is made up of permeable energy fields. The quantum healer attempts to work with these energy fields in order to enhance healing and bring back a sense of equilibrium. So, too, does the shaman, who tries to harmonize the energies that exist within the person affected by illness and between that person and the wider spiritual world. In both cases, the practitioner induces an altered state of consciousness in order to access deeper levels of awareness and facilitate healing.

A hallmark of shamanism is the use of ritual and symbol to deepen intention and amplify energy. Objects associated with specific healing functions might be feathers, stones, or drums—living forms endowed with spiritual qualities that focus healing energies with their inherent symbolic significance. Drawing on similar practices, quantum healing techniques utilize visualization, intention-setting, and energetic tools to influence the quantum field in support of therapeutic aims.

Furthermore, both shamanism and quantum healing also place great emphasis on the consciousness of the healer and the energy of intentionality. The shaman's ability to enter the spiritual realms and direct the healing energy is key to successful results in shamanism. Likewise, the practitioner's intent and consciousness are crucial in quantum healing when directing energy to influence the energy fields for healing.

Ultimately, it is this notion, that health and illness are fundamentally tied to the state of one's energy field, that may be the core commonality between shamanism and quantum healing. This energy field can, in altered states of consciousness, be accessed and brought into balance, thus restoring the seeker's health and well-being.

When this happens, it is said that a person can be so deeply shamanized or quantumized that they'll never be the same again. What quantum healing and shamanism together represent is a return to a holistic approach to health that transcends the narrower and often misguided world views of our modern era and gets back to the humanist roots of ancient wisdom, which viewed a person as more than just their body, brain, or heart.

Reiki (Japan)

Reiki and quantum healing are rooted in the idea that health and wellness are directly correlated with the movement of energy through and in the body. Persons attending to their health through quantum healing seek to resonate their body in such a way that it "rings" at precisely the correct frequency; likewise, the goal of a Reiki treatment session is to ensure that life-force energy has no impediments as it flows through the body so that it can self-heal.

The analogy with quantum healing is clear: If a practitioner can tap into healing energy fields and direct them to the patient, according to quantum healing, vibrational energy fields that are out of balance or unhealthy can be recovered. The healing of energy blocks and the harmonizing of the body occur as the energy is enhanced and flow restored. Similarly, in Reiki, universal life force energy is transferred to the patient and directed to the points where it is blocked or unbalanced.

One of the fundamental ideas of Reiki is that the practitioner should evolve into an open and attentive conduit for universal energy. Similarly, one of the key components of quantum healing is the notion that healing can result from a targeting of intention and consciousness onto the quantum field.

It is characteristic of Reiki's healing approach that its practitioners and their patients are encouraged to engage in disciplines that promote a positive mental attitude, coupled with an openness to feelings of compassion and their unity with the universal life force. This emphasis on whole-being involvement and the animating power of consciousness matches the ethos of quantum healing, albeit without embracing its radical physics.

The efficacy of both these modalities stems from the ability of the healers' hands to channel healing energy and direct it to the parts of the person who need to be healed to restore balance to their energetic and psychological life. The combination of ancient spiritual healing practices and modern science offers a holistic health strategy that makes us look at health from a new perspective going beyond the allopathic paradigm.

Yoga (India)

The parallels between yoga and quantum healing are easy to see.

The four pillars of quantum healing are indispensable elements in yoga too:

- Energy flow
- Body and mind
- Thought
- Action

The goal of yoga is the proper alignment of the body in asanas and the regulation of breath in pranayama, both designed to maximize the energy system of the body.

Meditation is an equally crucial element in both yoga and quantum healing. In yoga, it helps induce a state of serenity and heightened awareness. In quantum healing, meditation enables the mind and consciousness to influence the body's energy fields and thereby restore health.

Furthermore, there is awareness in both yoga and quantum healing that people have a body-mind-spirit system. Yoga has long been a holistic practice of health, seeking balance both within the physical body and the mental/emotional and spiritual bodies. Quantum healing also seeks body, mind, and spirit balance, combining intentional work with both the physical system and the energy systems encoded in the body.

A more direct way in which yoga can work with the body's quantum field is through the practice of yoga itself. Yoga may promote its own healing by relaxing the body, reducing stress, and improving the flow of prana, as every yoga practitioner knows. Research reveals that these benefits include decreased cortisol levels, improved immune function, and increased feelings of vitality. All of these are key aspects of a quantum healing practice that works to adjust the body's energy frequencies to the optimal setting for health and healing.

Overall, there are similarities between the practice of yoga, with physical and breathing exercises and meditation, and quantum healing. Both say that energy is fundamental to medicine because your body is constantly out of energy and who you are is the integration of your body and energy. Doing yoga, using breath, and doing meditation on a regular basis is the only way we can rebalance our system with gravity, so it works perfectly. Yoga works with quantum anatomy, neuroanatomy, and physiology. In this way, practicing yoga regularly will lead to profound and lasting positive changes, helping you achieve your deepest desires and goals by aligning your body and energy in harmony.

Sufism (Islamic Mysticism)

What quantum healing shares with Sufism is the sheer force of intention and belief, or, as Sufis have long known, *the truth of the heart and intention are close to God, and far from Him are the truth of the tongue and the hearing of the ears.*

In Sufism, spiritual communities concentrate their intentions and prayers on the immediate needs of their mentally ill members, invoking God's direct intervention. Similarly, quantum healers know that where the mind directs its focus, energy from the environment will likely be drawn to the site of that focus—a belief resonant with the Quran's language that calls upon the believing faithful.

Just as quantum healing practitioners visualize specific places or objects and direct healing energy fields, Sufis use intensive methods of *zikr* (chanted remembrance of God) to create harmonic connections with more subtle and spiritual energies. Practitioners in both traditions believe that the world of our senses is only a thin layer of reality that we must surpass, applying our full mental engagement to penetrate to a more substantial and energetic realm.

Similarly, Sufism teaches the healing power of love and compassion. Both Sufism and quantum healing philosophy confirm that positive emotions and thoughts can have a profound effect on health. The Sufi path of love, in which the lover surrenders self to the beloved, mirrors quantum healing's focus on shifting one's consciousness toward a more positive, harmonious state to attract good health.

Moreover, Sufism and quantum healing share the dogmatic belief in a universal energy or divine presence that permeates all matter. For the former, this energy is Allah; for the latter it is the quantum field or universal energy. Though the language differs, the desire to attune to the universal energy harbors in both traditions the hope of achieving higher states of consciousness and wellness.

Both Sufism and quantum healing have a robust notion of the spiritual realm emanating its energy to an energetic body on a fundamental level as well as the extraordinary transformative powers that spiritual practices can produce in them. Through meditation, chanting, self-reflection, and contemplation of love and compassion, both of these traditions aim to connect with a universal energy, energy field, or cosmic consciousness through which one can achieve spiritual salvation and holistic wellness.

Distinctive Healing Traditions: A Quick Overview

- **Ayurveda (India):** Balance—Focuses on balancing the body's three doshas (Vata, Pitta, and Kapha) to maintain health and prevent illness.
- **Traditional Chinese Medicine (TCM) (China):** Energy Flow—Emphasizes the flow of Qi (vital energy) through the body's meridians, using acupuncture, herbal medicine, and other techniques.
- **Shamanism (Global Indigenous Cultures):** Ritual and Journey—Uses rituals, trance, and spiritual journeys to heal and restore balance between the physical and spiritual worlds.
- **Reiki (Japan):** Universal Energy—Involves channeling universal life force energy through the hands to promote healing and balance in the recipient's energy field.

- **Yoga (India):** Integration of Body and Energy—Combines physical postures, breath control, and meditation to harmonize the body's energy and improve overall well-being.
- **Sufism (Islamic Mysticism):** Spiritual Transformation—Seeks a deep personal connection with the divine through practices like meditation, chanting, and asceticism to purify the soul and achieve spiritual enlightenment.

Next Steps

We have barely scraped the surface of quantum healing and a lot more is needed. But we have finally arrived at a point of intimate contact between ancient wisdom and modern science. Through Ayurveda, traditional Chinese medicine, shamanism, Sufism, and other traditions, we are embarking on a moment of integration that is long-awaited and well-met.

The similarities of intent between many of these ancient traditions and quantum healing point to the universal truth that healing is our nature. It comes from the energy that spins in and around us. Thus, this exploration of world religions and their ancient wisdom allows us to begin with a broader knowledge base. This includes learning how we as observers have an effect on the universe; the principles of quantum entanglement, superposition, and the observer effect; and practical exercises for energy balancing, meditation, and visualization.

Embodiment of these principles will allow you to utilize quantum healing and transform by embracing the vibrant consciousness of our multi-dimensional quantum universe. In the next chapter, you will learn the practical steps of becoming a certified quantum healer that will enable you to step up and help make the world a better place through the use of your healing arts.

REFERENCES

1. Eliade, M. (1964). *Shamanism: Archaic Techniques of Ecstasy*. Princeton University Press.
2. Goleman, D. (2006). *Emotional Intelligence*. Bantam Books.
3. Harner, M. (1980). *The Way of the Shaman*. Harper & Row.
4. Kabat-Zinn, J. (1994). *Wherever You Go, There You Are: Mindfulness Meditation in Everyday Life*. Hyperion.
5. Kaptchuk, T. J. (2000). *The Web That Has No Weaver: Understanding Chinese Medicine*. McGraw-Hill.
6. Lad, V. (2002). *Ayurveda: The Science of Self-Healing*. Lotus Press.
7. Lipton, B. H. (2005). *The Biology of Belief: Unleashing the Power of Consciousness, Matter & Miracles*. Hay House.
8. Maciocia, G. (2005). *The Foundations of Chinese Medicine: A Comprehensive Text for Acupuncturists and Herbalists*. Churchill Livingstone.
9. Miles, P., & True, G. (2003). "Reiki—Review of a Biofield Therapy: History, Theory, Practice, and Research." Alternative Therapies in Health and Medicine, 9(2), 62–72.
10. Myss, C. (1997). *Anatomy of the Spirit: The Seven Stages of Power and Healing*. Harmony.
11. Rand, W. L. (1998). *Reiki: The Healing Touch*. Vision Publications.
12. Svoboda, R. E. (1992). *Ayurveda: Life, Health, and Longevity*. Penguin Books.
13. Weiss, B. L. (2004). *Many Lives, Many Masters: The True Story of a Prominent Psychiatrist, His Young Patient, and the Past-Life Therapy That Changed Both Their Lives*. Simon & Schuster.

9
Becoming a Certified Quantum Healer

*"To become a healer, you must first heal yourself.
The journey of self-discovery and mastery is the
foundation of any true healing practice."*
—Dr. Mikao Usui

UNDERSTANDING THE FUNDAMENTALS

If you've read this far, congratulations! You're serious about becoming a quantum healer, and I commend you for your dedication. Your commitment to learning these principles is an essential step on your journey to becoming a proficient and compassionate healer. This path requires both knowledge and heart, and by diving into these basics, you're preparing yourself to make a significant impact on the well-being of others. Let's embark on this next crucial phase of your journey together and I'll make sure you get started on the right foot.

In the last chapter, we explored various healing traditions and the potential they hold. Now, in this chapter, we will focus specifically on quantum healing and some valuable resources you can use to train. Before you can become certified as a quantum healer, there are some basics you absolutely need to know and understand. You will need to master what the quantum healing paradigm is all about and what supports it in the broad context of holistic health practices. This chapter will outline the basics you need and what's required to know in order to be an effective quantum healer.

Quantum Entanglement

Quantum healing embodies the notion that the human body is connected; each part inseparably entangled with the others and with the universal energy field. As entangled photons are always connected no matter how far apart they end up, so, too, are the various manifestations of our physical, mental, and energetic bodies.

This level of connection and interconnectedness suggests not only that changes in one part of the body can instantaneously impact another but also that it is the sum of what works together that is of primary focus. One particular aspect of what works in a healthy body might be out of alignment while other aspects are functioning as normal. To approach wellness in this context means focusing both on the entangled aspects in need of repair, as well as, and more importantly, on harmonizing and balancing the whole rather than constructing patches for broken parts.

Quantum Superposition

Quantum superposition posits that a particle can be both in state A and state B simultaneously, until it is observed or measured. The best-known example of this principle is the thought experiment devised by Schrödinger, the cat in a box, which can be both dead and alive simultaneously until someone opens the box to observe it.

Thus, the phenomenon of superposition enables quantum healers to understand that health unfolds not in just one way but in a myriad of potential forms, depending on the intentions, observations, and consciousness of the healer and patient. By acting as a beacon or lens, a quantum healer can energize the system toward its optimal ground state. By harvesting positive intentions and the power of consciousness, quantum healers attempt to help bodies heal toward their optimal ground states.

Energy and Vibrational Frequencies

As we've previously discussed, everything in the universe, including the body, is literally energy in vibrational form. In other words, matter is energy. Ancient healing traditions, such as energy medicine, take for granted that if the correct vibration is not kept up, health will decline.

Energy healing is about boosting these vibrations in order to create health. Practitioners of quantum healing employ sound therapy and Reiki, along with a vast array of other energy healing modalities, to help rebalance body frequencies with what we have learned are beneficial, healthy frequencies.

Through sound therapy, Reiki, and other energy healing modalities, the aim of the energy healer often involves "tuning in" to the body and returning health to the body through an alignment with healthy, harmonious, and proper frequencies that lack dissonance, imbalance, and disharmony. In this way, those practices can help restore body processes to a healthy state for self-healing.

The Observer Effect

Just by measuring or looking at something, that thing is altered. This is often discussed in terms of the so-called observer effect, which says that measurement influences the phenomenon by observing it.

In the quantum field of healing, the observer effect validates the potential of consciousness and intention to heal and transform. Intention, prayer, and loving consciousness from a healer and the patient can directly impact the flow of energy of the body system, which can in turn facilitate healing by connecting to the energy field of mind and heart.

This means that if you change your thoughts, you can literally change your physical world. The same idea also suggests a role for a practitioner's or patient's can-do approach to healing, which has a direct effect on their attitude and disposition. A mindful, positive, focused, and intentionally hopeful perception can help facilitate profound health and healing, bestowing huge power over one's personal growth and well-being through the observer effect.

Integrating These Concepts

Understanding these core principles and ideas offers a glimpse into why and how quantum healing works. It explains how the ideas of connectedness, potentiality, and consciousness of the observer all come together. All of these are intrinsic to health and present a powerful way of thinking about and practicing healing.

I know this might seem like a lot of information, but it's not so complicated when you put these principles into practice. In fact, you can see these principles present in ancient traditions as well, reflecting timeless wisdom that aligns perfectly with modern scientific discoveries. As more of these ideas are tested and integrated into practice, the horizon of possibilities for transformative healing will only expand.

These ideas are not only astrological but also and at the same time pre-scientific and modern. Embracing them can help bridge the gap between ancient wisdom and contemporary science, allowing us to unlock new potentials for healing and well-being.

INTRODUCTORY MATERIALS, BOOKS, AND RESOURCES

Advancing along the certified quantum health career track requires an immersive, far-reaching training program supplemented by educational material that teaches you the ins and outs of the method, the skills, and the theoretical principles that will support and even define your journey. This section introduces some books, online courses, and workshops that can act as a first step toward a continued, all-encompassing, engagement with quantum healing.

The Field by Lynne McTaggart: This comprehensive guide to the science of the quantum field and its implications for understanding the universe and healing rocketed to the top of the New Age bestseller lists, earning accolades and an army of admirers. In this book, McTaggart cites scientific work and their anecdotes that most resonated with her own. She features the Zero Point Field, which underlies and holds every bit of the universe together, and claims it could be the key to all so-called psychic or spiritual phenomena, including telepathy, healing, and other paranormal abilities. By popularizing esoteric scientific theory for a general audience, McTaggart ensures that she can show those who pick up her book and apply themselves to the craft of reading how quantum theory might play a role in the healing arts.

Quantum-Touch: The Power to Heal **by Richard Gordon:** Richard Gordon, whom I mentioned in Chapter 2, explains in his book the technique used in his Quantum-Touch energy healing sessions. He describes his designation as a healer as "a technology for harnessing the healing energy of the body and focusing that energy to maximize the body's ability to heal itself."

The book specifically describes the technique and use of a specific breathing method and body awareness exercises to allow you to focus and release more healing energy. The book also presents detailed instructions and illustrations on how to use the energy. Gordon's clear explanations and case studies provide insight into the different conditions the technique can address by making the effectiveness of Quantum-Touch applicable and practical.

Workshops and Seminars: There are many workshops and seminars for practitioners to further explain the various aspects of energy medicine and quantum healing, given by those who are experienced healers, scientists, and educators. Workshops often focus on specific modalities such as Reiki, pranic healing, and advanced meditation techniques. These can be very beneficial, and many people who are interested in the field of energy medicine and quantum healing sign up for them. They would include hands-on practice with expert instructors. I have been teaching seminars for over two decades that focus on healing, health, and several different modalities as I describe above. I include lectures, demonstrations, and any manner of hands-on activities for attendees. These also allow you to network with fellow practitioners and gain a deeper understanding of the latest research and development in quantum healing.

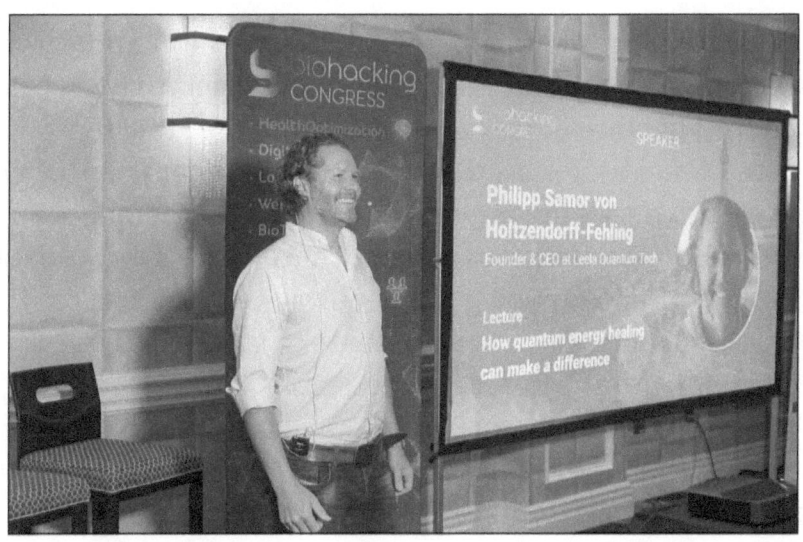

Speaking at the Biohacking Conference in Las Vegas in 2022.

EDUCATION AND TRAINING PROGRAMS

Along your journey to becoming a quantum healing practitioner, you undertake formal education and rigorous training that provide you with the required knowledge, skills, and connections to a community of quantum healers composing a broad spectrum destined to bring about a "quantum shift" in healing.

Certified Quantum Energy Practitioner Course

The Certified Quantum Energy Practitioner course from Leela Quantum Tech is a helpful training choice for aspiring quantum healers and is one of the most comprehensive programs available. I highly recommend it, but I might be a bit biased since I helped develop it! This course incorporates not just theoretical education but some practical lessons as well.

The training addresses developing intuition and setting intentions, as well as how to visualize and observe subtle fields of energy, balance those fields, and strengthen their flow. The course covers materials that will help you meet your own or your clients' needs for different types of healing. It ranges from the purely fundamental to more advanced topics for students who have already made good headway with the basics. This course is ideal for anyone who wants to study this topic from scratch or learn the latest techniques.

The Certified Quantum Energy Practitioner training is among the most notable teaching programs for quantum healing, with its comprehensive offering of material that is both theoretical and applied. It ensures participants gain a deep understanding of how to best apply quantum healing methods.

Here's an overview of what to expect when you enroll in the course.

Principles of Quantum: A thorough examination and understanding of the principles of quantum are an essential starting point for quantum healing. While these principles can be complex, they are the basis for everything that takes place through quantum healing. Once the basics are covered, participants will be sensitized to the ways in which these quantum principles can be utilized in their work.

Energy Balancing: Coursework involves intensive training in various techniques of energy balancing. These include techniques for maintaining and restoring optimal energetic balance as an essential aspect of a lifestyle conducive to physical, emotional, and spiritual health. The course offerings include Reiki, pranic healing, and the use of quantum devices for balancing energy fields.

Mastering and Using Quantum Devices: One of the unique attributes of Leela Quantum Tech is that it trains students to use quantum devices. It expounds on the science behind the devices and teaches students to incorporate use of the tools into their healing practices.

Practical Sessions: Trainees will gain quantum healing experience through hands-on practical sessions to apply the training and develop the skills they've learned. The course focuses on several topic areas, including the art of energy sensing, working with intentions, honing intuition, and manipulating energy flows with the chakras.

Ethical Training and Professional Preparedness: Trainees learn how to ensure that quantum healing is conducted responsibly and ethically. They are taught to develop respect for the wisdom life holds, recognize and appreciate their clients' autonomy and choices, observe professional boundaries, and respect confidentiality.

Holistic Approach: The holistic nature of the Certified Quantum Energy Practitioner training empowers graduates to understand the broad framework of healing including body, mind, and spirituality as one. A balanced approach to quantum healing with both time-honored wisdom of the ancients and modern-day scientific advancements is the key to facilitating true healing.

Graduates of the Leela Quantum Tech program are trained to the highest standards, poised to enter the field of quantum healing as knowledgeable practitioners who offer energy-healing services and client-centered sessions while utilizing new and groundbreaking quantum technologies to promote healing on all levels of mental, emotional, energetic, and physical being.

OTHER REPUTABLE INSTITUTIONS

Several other reputable organizations also offer formal training in energy medicine and quantum healing methods. Whether you're interested in learning these techniques through an online program or an in-person workshop, you have options that can fit your schedule and learning style.

Quantum University

Quantum University offers a range of courses in integrative medicine and energy healing. You can start with an associate's degree in Quantum Healing and work your way up to a Quantum Doctorate, achieving a Mastery of Health Transformation at each degree level. As anyone who has examined the science of quantum healing knows, it's essential for adherents of the practice to have a strong foundation in the life sciences.

The curriculum at Quantum University lets quantum healers integrate the ancient spiritual practices of healing, which have lent long-standing healing mythologies their weight and power, with modern scientific understandings.

Quantum University offers bachelor's, master's, and doctorate degree programs, as well as certification courses that cover all aspects of quantum healing. The curriculum is a rigorous blend of academic coursework and practical hands-on training, which helps students develop the skills needed to become a quantum healer for a professional practice. Students get the opportunity to apply their theoretical knowledge in clinical internships, workshops, and supervised practice sessions under the guidance of expert mentors.

When you sign up for a course at Quantum University, you are also joining an online social network where you can "friend" other people, both students and graduates, to network, discuss their research, and offer support. Through community-building, Quantum University alleviates some of the isolation that quantum healing practitioners can feel as they walk a path that isn't especially well-traveled.

Cru von Holtzendorff-Fehling

Born with the ability to see aura and energy fields, Cru has established a whole training series that not only enables you to truly get to know yourself and your inner essence in a very deep way but also enables you to see energy patterns, move through energy blockages, see the root cause of problems energetically, and become more comfortable in helping others. Her training series includes a variety of courses, one of which, the Path of Purification, is led by Cru and me together. This specific course isn't as much about helping others heal but about healing yourself and reestablishing a deep and conscious connection to the divine, to your true inner essence. You can find out more on Cru's website, cru-essence.com.

The Healing Touch Program

The Healing Touch Program provides a structured curriculum specific to energy therapy techniques, aimed at balancing and realigning the human energy system. An early and ongoing proponent of providing a structured, systematic learning pathway to energy work and healing, Healing Touch offers a variety of curricula available in these techniques and methods, including chakra balancing, aura cleansing, distance healing, and the power of the mind/healer's intent to focus and direct energy.

The Healing Touch Program's certification path includes a series of levels. To be certified at a particular tier, individuals need to complete the previous tier's training course. This means that every succeeding level builds on the previous tier of training.

In the first three levels of training in Healing Touch, the focus is on building a foundation in energy medicine. This includes learning about the human energy system and the corresponding basic healing techniques. Once students have experienced monochronic energy healing, they are introduced to more complex—or perhaps, polychronic—approaches to energy medicine in subsequent levels of training. Techniques such as working with specific conditions and using healing energy to address emotional and spiritual disturbances are taught in these higher levels.

ONLINE PLATFORMS AND WORKSHOPS

Many websites, such as Udemy, Coursera, and the Institute of Integrative Quantum Medicine offer online quantum healing courses for those interested in exploring this subject. The quantum sphere of education varies from beginner to advanced.

Online Options

Popular online course site Udemy sells several courses on quantum healing, which learners can engage in from the comfort of their own homes and at their own pace. These courses include video lectures, reading material, and various exercises.

In some cases, learners are even assigned homework that can be completed at their own discretion. In one of these courses, students can expect to learn the fundamentals of energy healing, as well as how to use energy from the quantum field for the purpose of healing. Such courses are often created by practitioners and teachers with years of experience in the field.

Coursera, a massive open online course (MOOC) platform, offers courses in quantum healing and related topics, some in collaboration with universities and research institutes. The courses review the science more deeply by delving into the biofield, biofield science, the neuroscience of healing, and practical applications of quantum principles in the medical and therapeutic contexts. They contain peer-reviewed assignments, quizzes, and opportunities to collaborate with other students on a forum. The time frame is structured and students receive a certification from renowned institutions after completing the courses.

The Institute of Integrative Quantum Medicine offers specialized courses on integrating quantum principles within classical and modern healing practices. This includes training in advanced quantum neurofeedback as well as energy field modulation and the therapeutic use of quantum devices.

In addition to offering an academic education, the course claims to train the individual from a very practical level with the use of devices to improve one's quality of life, including reducing degenerative illnesses. In line with quantum medicine, the institute not only offers courses but also guarantees that its students continue to pursue investigative research for as long as they are associated with the institute, including through ongoing mentorship programs.

Hands-On Workshops

Quantum healing workshops are intensive training programs conducted online or in person for a few days or a few weeks. They are suitable for hands-on learners.

Workshops generally have interactive teaching sessions and practical demonstrations, and they offer opportunities for learners to practice techniques on one another, with the ability to receive feedback from instructors. These workshops specifically deal with specialized quantum tools of healing energy and provide in-depth training in their respective domains.

Followers of the online workshops are able to log on, regardless of location in the world, while the in-person workshops provide a small but concentrated community of learners directly confined to the location of the event.

Both forms of providing this instruction to the masses are equally valuable, particularly as they offer the possibility for people to find out what works best for them, allowing learners to pick and choose between modes of instruction that free them from an imposed education model. Ultimately, this will provide any future quantum healers with a strong skill set equipped with the knowledge and experiences to enter the world of energy medicine.

Pursuing Certification

Being certified through a program will provide you with a stamp of approval and a community of fellow quantum healers to serve as a reference to your abilities. Assessments, practical testing, and continuing education are often requirements of certification programs, in part, to help ensure the practitioner maintains their proficiency and is up to date. Programs provide community, lifelong learning, and opportunities for networking.

One of the most invaluable aspects of my own journey was the community of quantum healers I became a part of. The support, shared experiences, and collective wisdom of this community were instrumental to my growth and development. I cannot emphasize enough how much a community can help navigate the complexities and challenges of becoming a proficient healer.

Follow these steps and you will be on your way to becoming a certified quantum healer. This powerful new process will give you and those you help the tools to have broad and deep impacts on the health of others. You will have access to ancient wisdom and modern science that teaches new ways of understanding the mind-body connection and exploring the power of human consciousness to create a quantum shift in healing.

REFERENCES

1. Bohm, D. (1980). *Wholeness and the Implicate Order*. Routledge.
2. Einstein, A., Podolsky, B., & Rosen, N. (1935). "Can Quantum-Mechanical Description of Physical Reality Be Considered Complete?" *Physical Review*, 47(10), 777–780. https://doi.org/10.1103/PhysRev.47.777.
3. Gerber, R. (2001). *Vibrational Medicine: The #1 Handbook of Subtle-Energy Therapies*. Bear & Company.
4. Gordon, R. (2006). *Quantum-Touch: The Power to Heal*. North Atlantic Books.
5. Grof, S., & Grof, C. (2010). *Holotropic Breathwork: A New Approach to Self-Exploration and Therapy*. State University of New York Press.
6. Kaptchuk, T. J. (2000). *The Web That Has No Weaver: Understanding Chinese Medicine*. McGraw-Hill.

7. Leela Quantum Tech. (2025). Certified Quantum Energy Practitioner Course.

8. McTaggart, L. (2008). *The Field: The Quest for the Secret Force of the Universe*. Harper Perennial.

9. Miles, P., & True, G. (2003). "Reiki—Review of a Biofield Therapy: History, Theory, Practice, and Research." *Alternative Therapies in Health and Medicine*, 9(2), 62–72.

10. National Center for Complementary and Integrative Health. (2018, December). "Reiki." U.S. Department of Health and Human Services, National Institutes of Health. https://www.nccih.nih.gov/health/reiki.

11. Quantum University. (n.d.). Integrative Medicine and Energy Healing Programs. https://quantumuniversity.com/.

12. Schrödinger, E. (1935). "Die gegenwärtige Situation in der Quantenmechanik." *Die Naturwissenschaften*, 23(48), 807–812.

10
Future Possibilities

*"The future belongs to those who believe
in the beauty of their dreams."*
—Eleanor Roosevelt

Quantum healing is holistic and reaches the body's energy fields. This means that in addition to manifesting as specific physical issues, it has great potential as a holistic complement to any kind of medical therapy. There are different ways of integrating quantum healing into mainstream healthcare.

Integration involves blending the energetic principles of quantum healing with traditional medical treatments to provide a more complete way of attaining better health. One way is to include energetic balancing exercise in patient care. Another is to use quantum healing as an adjunctive therapy on top of conventional treatments. A third approach is to train doctors and other healthcare professionals in the fundamentals of quantum and energy healing.

BENEFITS OF INTEGRATION

People often report that the combination of conventional medicine treatments and quantum healing treatments leads to quicker recovery. More obvious benefits include improved health outcomes, such as better control of chronic conditions, improved quality of life, increased patient satisfaction, and more.

Compelling Evidence and Case Studies

Several case studies and journal articles outline the successful integration of quantum healing into mainstream medical care. For example, work published in the *Journal of Oncology Nursing* examined Reiki as a complementary cancer therapy for patients undergoing chemotherapy. Their findings indicated that Reiki decreased reported levels of pain, anxiety, and fatigue in these patients compared with those who did not receive Reiki. This suggests that Reiki is a useful auxiliary therapy in a standard cancer care regimen.

Analogously, an article on acupuncture and post-surgical recovery in the *Frontiers in Medicine* found that patients who underwent knee replacement surgery who were then treated with acupuncture showed significant function improvement and a lower percentage of nausea/vomiting in comparison with the groups who underwent standard post-operative care.

Enhancing Treatments with a Holistic Approach

Quantum healing, which focuses on the energy fields of the body and on "wellness" as the goal of healing, is a complementary approach to encouraging the body's natural and inner processes to heal. What would quantum healing look like integrated into "mainstream" medical care?

It would function as a more holistic (or comprehensive) and possibly more effective approach to health. For instance, let's say you know you need an invasive surgery of some kind—which, by the way, is okay. While I view quantum healing as helpful and even as a form of medicine, using quantum healing does not at all mean that other needed forms of medicine should be shunned. It simply means that upon diagnosis, in addition to the treatment plan for the invasive surgery, you could also base your treatment plan on quantum healing.

In this instance, an important advantage of adding quantum healing to modern medicine and seeking to supplement the more classic approach mentioned earlier could be the reduction of side effects caused by post-surgery issues. These kinds of practices as a complement to conventional medical treatments support the human body's capacity for self-repair—in excess of what might be expected based on medications and procedures alone.

This includes lower incidences of complications and can translate into shorter hospital stays, reduced insurance costs, and faster recuperative times. When it comes to chronic illnesses, patients who choose a joint treatment find their conditions effectively managed, experience better outcomes in their overall health, and obtain an increased sense of satisfaction with their experiences in the healthcare system.

Paving the Way for Unified Healing

For these reasons, the vision of quantum healing being fully integrated with mainstream medical care seems poised to create significant improvements in patient care and overall health outcomes. It combines the best of both healing traditions in a way that allows doctors and other healthcare providers to better serve and honor those in their care. Via further research, and as more case studies and journal articles highlight the benefits of integrating quantum healing practices into mainstream healthcare, our quantum medicine future will emerge into the present, becoming fully accepted and implemented in hospitals and clinics across the globe.

ADVANCEMENTS IN DEVICES AND TECHNOLOGIES

The future of quantum healing looks promising, especially as new devices and technologies are constantly being developed with the goal of expanding its applications even further.

More advanced versions of biofeedback devices, which provide real-time feedback on physiological functions, could be developed to monitor and alter the energy profile of a living being. Based on these readings, it might soon be possible to address issues directly based on an individual's idiosyncratic energetic balance, facilitating healing like never before.

Another potentially beneficial innovation is energy field scanners. Practitioners would be able to view the patient's different energy fields, evaluate their imbalances, and see where external energy fields could be applied. The scientific community is also researching various quantum sensors and imaging technologies, aiming to develop accurate and reliable energy field scanners. For example, studies of heart rate variability (HRV) biofeedback have already demonstrated reductions in stress and improvements in autonomic function. It is reasonable to assume that future advances could harness quantum principles to boost biofeedback's therapeutic potential even further.

Eventually, smart health-promoting environments might exist. Such environments would adapt their energies to those of their inhabitants, possibly using sensors, algorithms, and smart quantum technologies, to aid in general wellness and health. As one example, an energy-field-modulating smart home could automatically keep its occupants in excellent health by adapting the color, light, and darkness of its rooms, as well as room temperature and electromagnetic fields, in accordance with inhabitants' internal energy environment.

These technologies could be widely implemented in future clinics for practitioners to use in patient revitalization and vitality enhancement. This could eventually even draw together traditional medicine and wellness therapies as a single discipline.

Generally speaking, the combination of quantum healing with conventional medicine, supported by innovative devices and technologies, will open up the vast potential for human healing in the near future. By leveraging the strength of both methods, quantum health practitioners can provide more complete and effective treatments when providing holistic healthcare.

PERSONALIZED HEALING JOURNEYS

Just as personalized medicine, which addresses a patient's genetics, lifestyles, and environmental factors, is the new standard of care, personalized quantum healing will similarly strive for the greatest benefit for a particular patient, based on their individual energy signature.

The process of personalized medicine starts with an assessment of a patient's unique energy patterns. Ayurvedic medicine identifies seven types of body-energy patterns, and quantum healing aligns each patient's healing approach with the specific energetic frequencies that make that individual a unique energy field. In this way, quantum healing treatment is completely tailored to the needs of each person. Just as modern medical doctors tailor treatment according to an individual body's genetic propensities, quantum healing customizes its treatment to align with the individual's unique energy field.

Conducting Energy Assessments

Imagine a future where conducting an energy assessment transcends traditional methods, evolving into a seamless integration of technology and intuition.

It might be possible, for instance, for the healer to assess the energy field with a device that would provide biofeedback, which not only enables scanning the aura for information but also affords a minute-by-minute, detailed map of the energy field, showing where and how the energy is stuck, allowing healers to treat energy imbalances with much more precision.

In that future, healers might use quantum devices that sense tiny temperature changes, or shifts in electromagnetic fields, in order to gain a clearer and more holistic energetic picture rather than a purely intuitive one. In the future, these devices might even generate detailed reports that track anomalous energies over time, in ways that would help to develop a more flexible and adaptive treatment.

The longer-term speculative future of energy assessment could also involve personalized healing protocols. A healer could devise a unique healing protocol based on data from these cutting-edge assessments. A healer could use AI-driven insight and intuitive skill to create an individualized healing regimen, one that makes use of the patient's whole energetic profile and needs. Such a system could be much more effective at healing and would empower clients by giving them more knowledge about their energy fields and how to stay balanced.

In the longer term, this continued progress toward more efficient, finer-grained, and customized methods for assessing energy in the future will lead to better and more precise modes of healing. As technology and quantum healing continue to evolve, they will likely lead us to new horizons of energy, health, and the profound links between them.

Tips for Practitioners

If you are or aim to be a quantum energy healing practitioner, here's some food for thought as this field advances in the coming years.

Regular Energy Reassessments: Set up habitual energy assessments to track the client's progress and adjustments to the healing plan. This serves to confirm both the effectiveness and responsiveness of the treatment to a client's shifting needs.

Advanced Technologies: Use biofeedback devices and other advanced quantum healing technologies such as energy field scanners whose data can be sped up so you get real-time information about what is happening in the energy patterning.

Educate and Empower the Client: Teach the client about their energy signatures and educate them on how they can take the lead in their healing. Provide handouts and tools such as mindfulness or meditation practice that they can do between sessions to help maintain their energy balance.

Holistic Perspective: Don't lose the perspective that your work involves the entire being and organism. It's not just cysts and bone density tests. Encourage men and women to pursue related but non-medical paths—to do yoga, journal, meditate, and spend time outdoors.

If quantum healers can get in touch with the personalized energy signature of a client, they can engage in the personalized quantum healing process so that the quantum information can be put to effective use. The same is true of orthodox medicine. The 21st century psychophysiological revolution in medicine and health will ultimately hinge as much on our ability to engage personalized quantum healing with the energy signature of individuals as it will on conventional molecular approaches.

The Role of AI and Machine Learning

Given the rapid spread of artificial intelligence (AI) and machine learning into a variety of fields, including healthcare, it's only a matter of time until AI aids in the practice of quantum healing. By providing quantum healers with more precise, data-driven information about the energy fields in a patient's body, as well as more detailed understandings of the pathways to optimal health for that patient, AI has the potential to transform the practice of quantum healing for the better.

Quantum healing's AI algorithms can be trained to look at energy field data from sensors and devices to spot irregularities and disruptions in a client's energy field to a finer degree than traditional observation techniques allow. When practitioners start looking at data to inform their work, the precision of their healing efforts should improve through the quantum ability to integrate insights.

Another really exciting application of AI in quantum healing is in predicting effective healing paths. Machine learning models can easily examine large amounts of historical data collected from thousands of previous patients. What emerges are insights showing which healing techniques have been most effective on different categories of energy imbalances.

Current AI Applications in Healthcare

Although we have only a provisional idea of how AI could function as a healing tool, the integration of AI into healthcare is well underway, giving us a preview of its future potential. For example, algorithms analyze medical imaging to predict the progression of disease or determine the most suitable treatment regime based on composite features described in genetic data.

In oncology, researchers are already developing AI algorithms that learn patterns of tumor evolution and are able to recommend personalized treatment sequences. There are also AI-driven applications for mental health now emerging. For instance, mood disorders can be anticipated from the analysis of spoken language and behavior.

From there, it isn't hard to see how AI could be applied to interpret data from the quantum energy fields to help quantum healers become more precise in their work. Quantum health practitioners could gain a greater understanding of patients' illnesses, complement the skills of human healers, and even perform an initial triage of patients for more immediate inter-vention—all with the help of AI.

Future Developments in AI and Quantum Healing

Going forward, these two new technologies are set to evolve hand in hand. For example, advanced biofeedback devices with AI algorithms might monitor and shape the healing field of a human body in real time, informing a healer and a patient the instant their condition changed.

Moreover, AI could enable the creation of all-encompassing archives that collect data from thousands of quantum healing sessions, which could be analyzed by machine learning models through the aggregated data to uncover new correlations between energy patterns and health outcomes, pointing the way to even more new healing techniques and interventions.

Combining AI and machine learning with personalized quantum healing is the next logical step in the process. With the invention of quantum computers that will enable true machine learning, we will doubtless see more awesome breakthroughs in the industry. Quantum healing, in whatever form it evolves, will always be a holistic health practice, and it will lead us to better and more effective ways of healing the mind and body.

Global Consciousness Shift

We are on the cusp of a quantum healing revolution, as a spiritual-scientific boost to nutrition, the environment, and a holistic conception of wellness continues to gain influence each and every day. However, true planetary healing depends on individual human healing, and viceversa. This holistic understanding of health is becoming more widely accepted. It will play a major role in the emerging quantum healing revolution as the dangers of unhealthy living become increasingly obvious. We cannot overestimate the importance of understanding our interconnected place in the planetary organism.

The Hawkins Scale

Dr. David R. Hawkins's Map of Consciousness, often referred to as the Hawkins Scale, is a revolutionary framework that measures levels of human consciousness on a logarithmic scale from 1 to 1,000. This scale categorizes various states of consciousness, ranging from the lowest levels of shame and guilt to the highest states of enlightenment and pure consciousness. Hawkins's work emphasizes that these levels correspond to different attractor fields, which are energetic frequencies that shape our experiences and perceptions of reality.[1]

---

1   The ideas and concepts developed by Dr. Hawkins are used with the utmost respect and acknowledgment of his pioneering work in the field of consciousness studies. The interpretations and applications of these concepts in this book are the author's own and are meant to pay homage to Dr. Hawkins's groundbreaking research. The information derived from Dr. Hawkins's work is used under the principles of fair use for educational purposes and as a basis for further commentary and discussion. This book is an independent work and has not been endorsed by Dr. Hawkins or his estate. The discussion of these concepts in this book is intended to provide an interpretation and application of the ideas presented in Dr. Hawkins's research, aiming to further the discussion and understanding of consciousness in the context of personal and spiritual growth.

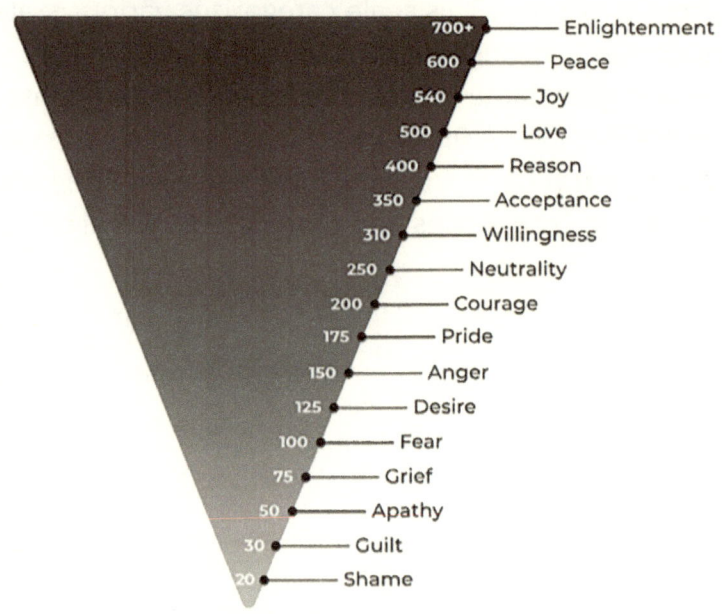

ULTIMATE CONSCIOUSNESS

700+	Enlightenment
600	Peace
540	Joy
500	Love
400	Reason
350	Acceptance
310	Willingness
250	Neutrality
200	Courage
175	Pride
150	Anger
125	Desire
100	Fear
75	Grief
50	Apathy
30	Guilt
20	Shame

The Map of Consciousness measures levels
of human consciousness on a scale.

Traditionally, Hawkins set the upper limit of the scale at 1,000, representing the pinnacle of human consciousness attainable during his time. However, advancements in consciousness and energy practices have since indicated that it's possible to access even higher levels. As our collective consciousness evolves, the vibrational capacity of individuals and objects can now surpass this original threshold.

Leela Quantum Tech and Quantum Upgrade are at the forefront of leveraging these higher levels of consciousness in their products and services. By calibrating their technologies at levels exceeding 2,200 on the Hawkins Scale, they harness higher frequencies that were previously unattainable. This breakthrough allows for more profound healing, greater balance, and enhanced well-being. It is also a strong indicator of what may be possible in the future.

Embracing Higher Consciousness in Quantum Healing

Quantum healing taps into these elevated states of consciousness to facilitate deeper healing processes. Here's how it works:

1. **Enhanced Vibrational States:** By using devices calibrated to higher levels on the Hawkins Scale, practitioners can access and channel stronger, more refined energies. This can lead to more effective healing sessions and better outcomes for clients.

2. **Improved Energy Flow:** Higher consciousness levels promote a smoother and more harmonious flow of energy within the body, helping to dissolve blockages and restore balance.

3. **Greater Resonance with Universal Energy:** Accessing higher vibrational frequencies aligns practitioners and clients with the universal energy fields, enhancing their ability to attract positive outcomes and experiences.

The Path Forward

Incorporating these advanced levels of consciousness into everyday practices and healing modalities signifies a significant shift in how we approach health and well-being. As more people and technologies align with these higher frequencies, we can expect a broader acceptance and integration of quantum healing principles into mainstream healthcare. This evolution holds the promise of transforming our individual lives and the collective consciousness, leading to a more harmonious and enlightened world.

By understanding and utilizing the Hawkins Scale, along-side cutting-edge technologies from Leela Quantum Tech and Quantum Upgrade, we are equipped to reach unprecedented levels of consciousness. This journey not only enhances personal growth but also contributes to the global shift toward higher awareness and interconnectedness.

Potential Risks and Ethical Considerations in Quantum Healing

Thus far, I've discussed the potential of quantum energy for healing, going into specific detail on the advantages it can bring. I think it's important, however, to take a brief look at the potential risks or downsides as well. I want to present a balanced discussion of quantum healing so you can have an informed opinion. For each potential risk, I also offer a proposed solution to help mitigate it.

Lack of Standardization

Standardization of quantum energy healing is perhaps its biggest risk. Currently, the field is unregulated. Practitioners have broad latitude over what they can use and how they use it. In the absence of stringent standards, quantum energy healing tools might be more or less effective, leading to a lack of confidence and trust among people considering whether to become a client as well as among conventional medical personnel.

Solution: A body of licensed quantum energy healing practices needs to be standardized. All practitioners will need to be certified, and the process for certification should be stringent and well-regulated. The curriculum should be developed collaboratively with existing medical organizations and professional bodies to facilitate the integration of quantum healing into regular medical practice.

Challenge in Quantifying Results

Another ongoing issue is the difficulty that comes with quantifying results. Quantum energy is an extremely subjective type of healing. That makes it very hard for people to move in that direction because it's not something that's been part of Western medicine for many, many years.

Solution: By embracing conventional medicine's testing procedures, those practitioners who adhere to quantum healing might have an easier time showing their approaches to people in power. Armed with data from controlled studies and clinical trials, quantum healers could begin to recapture the attention and, most importantly, the funds of physicians and insurance providers.

Religious and Cultural Considerations

Quantum healing can also run up against religious or cultural views and customs, limiting its ability to be embraced and integrated into diverse communities.

Solution: Recognition and understanding of these discrepancies are necessary. We need to standardize quantum healing to an extent that it is seen as part of regular medicine, not something you do in addition to regular medicine. For instance, we can design educational programs that explain what quantum healing is scientifically and how it fits into regular medicine to make it more acceptable to the regular audience.

Financial Risks

Quantum healing can be costly, and insurance usually doesn't cover it—meaning that those who might benefit most are prevented from accessing it because of a lack of funds.

Solution: For quantum healing to become mainstream, we will need proven results and standardization. We need to conduct testing and clinical trials to prove it works so insurance companies will start covering it. This will lower the cost burden for patients. Creating cost-effective technologies and techniques can help as well.

Ethical Considerations and Sustainability

In addition to the specific risks I have listed, there are also general ethical concerns and sustainability questions to consider. Practitioners should respect the privacy and confidentiality of their clients, ensure they are given informed consent about any quantum healing procedure, and not force them to undergo any treatment process unwillingly.

Another major ethical challenge is to ensure that quantum healing technologies are made available to all in an equitable manner so that the benefits of these technologies accrue to humanity as a whole. Otherwise, we run the risk of unequal distribution of quantum healing technologies, which has the potential to marginalize underserved communities once again.

Partnering with Public and Private Entities

Quantum healers may also partner with public or private entities on holistic public health projects. Quantum healers can team up with healthcare providers, educational institutions, or community organizations to design programs that integrate holistic practices into broader public health strategies. Such partnerships can help quantum healing become more widely accepted and understood.

Once these possible dangers and ethical concerns are addressed, quantum healing will be more readily accepted and incorporated into mainstream care. This will not only raise the profile of quantum healing but will also make it available to a much larger and more diverse audience, allowing for more balanced and holistic healthcare.

SUSTAINABLE HEALING FOR THE PLANET

These principles, originally applied only to humans in the context of health, could create the sustainable linkages needed through quantum ecology between the homeostasis of an individual organism and the homeostasis of the planet. This prompts us to consider some important questions. How can quantum healing create environmental sustainability? Can we envision huge energy field healing projects? What are the current sustainable practices in health?

Scale-up projects could apply quantum healing tactics to the restoration of ecological balance and the healing of environmental destruction across entire countries, regions, or continents. These projects could involve specific community-based rituals of meditation and intention-setting. For example, intentional communities could direct positive energy and intentions to global environmental issues such as deforestation, pollution, or climate change.

This could consist of many quantum healers synchronizing meditative intentions together to revitalize polluted water bodies or recharge exhausted soil. Essentially, imagine a global network of human energy that can synchronize and collectively share their prana with ecosystems in need. These collective efforts would be complemented by the appropriate presence of scientific monitoring and control measures.

Current Sustainable Practices in Healthcare

A number of sustainable practices in healthcare already conform to the tenets of quantum healing. This is especially the case with integrative medicine, where the objective is to combine conventional medical treatments with traditional and holistic approaches and procedures.

This often means a greater emphasis on environmental factors for health, leading integrative medicine to have a higher adherence to sustainable practices. For example, numerous treatments use organic and locally sourced materials to minimize their carbon footprint, and they have taken measures to become more energy-efficient in hospitals and surgical facilities.

Sustainable practices also include adopting green building standards for hospitals, with a view to reducing the carbon footprint of their operations and reducing waste. They also include using nature-based therapies, such as horticultural therapy and ecotherapy, in patient care, as part of a wider suite of therapies aiming to connect people with nature. These practices contribute to improved patient health outcomes and environmental health.

Future Applications of Quantum Healing

In the future, it would not be surprising to see quantum healing principles embraced by the green movement for its own interpretation of sustainability. Technologies that combine the informational energy fields of natural elements into a working device that heals and balances environmental concerns could be introduced. Devices that amplify the healing signals of plants and trees could be used by ecological restoration practitioners to revive degraded landscapes and whole ecosystems.

Another promising direction is biofeedback in combination with energy field scanners. With these, users could monitor the energetic health of ecosystems in real time. This would enable interventions designed to assist ecosystem healing and rejuvenation by supporting the energetic balance of the environment.

Quantum healing principles offer a unique and potentially powerful alternative approach to promoting environmentally friendly practices. If we imagine large-scale energy healing projects, implement integrative medicine and health programs with a focus on sustainability, and continually explore future applications, we can better leverage the flow of energy fields inherent in our universe and facilitate bringing back ecological and environmental harmony while healing the current ecological damage.

Initially considered pseudoscience, this approach offers the potential to bring about broader systemic changes by reinforcing the strong interconnectivity between our own health and the health of the ecosystem we exist in. The sooner we can develop and implement these practices, the sooner we can fully embrace the advent of quantum healing to enable the journey toward a sustainable and healthier world for all.

The Role of Community and Collaboration

What if quantum healers operated in a sprawling global network where they could interact across borders, bringing their respective quantum healing technologies to bear on the planet's collective problems? The expansion of digital communications in recent decades has meant that it is no longer impossible to envision a global network of quantum healers who could draw upon one another's knowledge, experience, and capacity to bring healing to the world's most pressing health problems on a planetary basis.

Let's say that an earthquake led to a variety of infrastructure issues in a given area. A global network of quantum psycho-therapists and energy healers could participate in a massive, transpersonal healing session over the planet to help people who are affected emotionally or physically in the ravaged region.

Social media and digital forums could help coordinate this worldwide cooperation. Using social media platforms, as well as specialized forums and websites, healers and those aiming to become quantum healers could find and read about one another's case studies, discuss new techniques, and provide one another with virtual workshops and sessions. In doing so, they would not only democratize access to quantum healing know-how but also build online communities connecting quantum healing practitioners all over the world.

Furthermore, quantum healers can host webinars, live Q&As, and collaborative research projects on digital platforms, allowing them to keep up with the latest developments in the field. Riding on social media, these networks can also introduce quantum healers to the general public, helping to expand the audience for the practice. Eventually, quantum healing might make its way into the realm of mainstream health practices.

Quantum healers could even begin to work with public or private institutions to provide holistic wellness services, expanding their reach and impact. This includes working with hospitals, schools, and community organizations to foster integrated wellness programs that offer both traditional medical and quantum healing approaches to health. This could help legitimize quantum healing by involving public institutions within this work, as well as help infuse public health with more balanced approaches to wellness. In this way, quantum healers and public institutions could work together to encourage the development of environments that foster health, ultimately helping to cultivate a culture of health that benefits us all.

REFERENCES

1. Bohm, D. (1980). *Wholeness and the Implicate Order*. Routledge.
2. Chen, Z., Shen, Z., Ye, X., Xu, Y., Liu, J., Shi, X., Chen, G., Wu, J., Chen, W., Jiang, T., Liu, W., & Xu, X. (2021). "Acupuncture for rehabilitation after total knee arthroplasty: A systematic review and meta-analysis of randomized controlled trials." *Frontiers in Medicine*, 7, 602564.
3. Chirico, A., D'Aiuto, G., Penon, A., Mallia, L., De Laurentiis, M., Lucidi, F., Botti, G., & Giordano, A. (2017). "Spiritual well-being in cancer patients: A randomized controlled trial." *Anticancer Research*, 37(7), 3657–3665.
4. Einstein, A., Podolsky, B., & Rosen, N. (1935). "Can Quantum-Mechanical Description of Physical Reality Be Considered Complete?" *Physical Review*, 47(10), 777–780.
5. Gerber, R. (2001). *Vibrational Medicine: The #1 Handbook of Subtle-Energy Therapies*. Bear & Company.
6. Gordon, R. (2006). *Quantum-Touch: The Power to Heal*. North Atlantic Books.
7. Grof, S., & Grof, C. (2010). *Holotropic Breathwork: A New Approach to Self-Exploration and Therapy*. State University of New York Press.
8. Kaptchuk, T. J. (2000). *The Web That Has No Weaver: Understanding Chinese Medicine*. McGraw-Hill.

9. Leela Quantum Tech. (2025). Quantum Energy Practitioner Introductory Course.

10. Lu, W., & Rosenthal, D. S. (2013). "Acupuncture for Cancer Pain and Related Symptoms." *Current Pain and Headache Reports*, 17(3), 321.

11. Manheimer, E., Cheng, K., Wieland, L. S., Min, L. S., Shen, X., Berman, B. M., & Lao, L. (2012). "Acupuncture for treatment of irritable bowel syndrome." *Cochrane Database of Systematic Reviews*, 2012(5), CD005111.

12. McTaggart, L. (2008). *The Field: The Quest for the Secret Force of the Universe*. Harper Perennial.

13. Miles, P., & True, G. (2003). "Reiki—Review of a Biofield Therapy: History, Theory, Practice, and Research." *Alternative Therapies in Health and Medicine*, 9(2), 62–72.

14. National Center for Complementary and Integrative Health. (2018, December). *"Reiki." U.S. Department of Health and Human Services, National Institutes of Health*. https://www.nccih.nih.gov/health/reiki.

15. Quantum University. (n.d.). *"Integrative Medicine and Energy Healing Programs."* https://quantumuniversity.com/.

16. Schrödinger, E. (1935). "Die gegenwärtige Situation in der Quantenmechanik." *Die Naturwissenschaften*, 23(48), 807–812.

17. Tsang, K. L., Carlson, L. E., & Olson, K. (2007). "Pilot Crossover Trial of Reiki Versus Rest for Treating Cancer-Related Fatigue." *Integrative Cancer Therapies*, 6(1), 25–35.

18. Vitale, A. T., & O'Connor, P. C. (2006). "The Effect of Reiki on Pain and Anxiety in Women with Abdominal Hysterectomies: A Quasi-Experimental Pilot Study." *Holistic Nursing Practice*, 20(6), 263–272.

Afterword

Now that we've come to the end of our time together, I invite you to reflect on how you have changed. After all, this book is more than a collection of knowledge; it's a portal that has opened your mind to deeper self-understanding and meaningful connections with the world at large. By exploring the principles of quantum healing, I hope you have grown and now relate to yourself and others in a healthier and more humane way. More importantly, I believe you've opened your mind, and perhaps your soul, to the view that all life is interconnected, traveling together on infinite waves of energy.

I celebrate the knowledge you have gained and the truths you have uncovered. This new level of awareness is not just your discovery but belongs to all who share the vision of quantum healing, a community that is continually growing. We are forging a new generation that sees health as encompassing physical, emotional, mental, and spiritual dimensions, and now you are a part of that journey.

Armed with this knowledge, it is time to lead the charge toward quantum health and support its integration into the mainstream healthcare systems to promote "holistic" health. This approach is the antidote to the current epidemic of toxicities, chaos, and disharmony. Advocate for holistic health and quantum healing concepts to be taught in educational curricula, cultivating future generations to remember our entangled existence and maintain energetic harmony and balance.

The best part? This is just the beginning. Quantum healing is a continually evolving field. Stay informed about new research, techniques, and technologies, and continue educating yourself in quantum healing. Be an active participant in the transformation of healing practices. Innovate and experiment to see how these principles can be applied in new ways. Your contributions, no matter how small, can help evolve the collective understanding, effectiveness, and proficiency of quantum healing.

To start, all we need to do is to visualize a world in which quantum healing principles have become part of mainstream thinking. A place where health is achieved not merely through the absence of disease but as a state of optimal dynamic balance of body, mind, heart, and spirit.

This joint vision allows us to realize our full potential as loving, compassionate, and joyful human beings. The world you envision—where energy flows freely, harmony prevails, and every living thing thrives—will be realized through the healing waters of new quantum medicine.

Thank you for joining me on this journey and for your openness to learning what Western medicine prefers to keep secret. Embracing quantum healing is a lifelong process. Trust in the journey and in yourself. Keep discovering, keep believing, and keep opening.

Wishing you blessings on your journey! May your path be illuminated with light, love, and boundless opportunities. Remember, together, we are transforming the world.

About the Author

Philipp Samor von Holtzendorff-Fehling is a coach, conscious entrepreneur, and energy healer whose journey bridges corporate leadership and holistic wellness. For years he held executive positions in Europe and the United States, including serving as Vice President at T-Mobile International and T-Mobile US. While building a successful business career, he trained extensively in shamanic and energy healing practices, past life regression, trauma therapy, and Kundalini yoga.

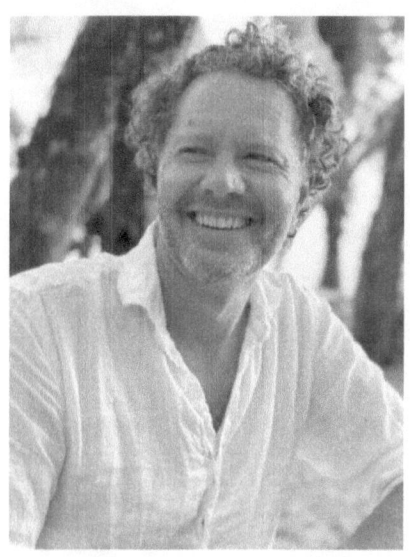

Philipp is the founder of Leela Quantum Tech and Quantum Upgrade, where he applies his expertise in quantum technology and frequency medicine to create tools that promote balance, vitality, and overall well-being. His unique ability to perceive energy fields, combined with decades of study in both ancient and modern approaches to healing, has made him a recognized leader in the field of energy work and quantum wellness.

In addition to his professional and healing work, Philipp is a dedicated athlete who became the number one ranked men's 50+ tennis player in the United States in 2024. He is also a devoted father and dog lover who values living with purpose, authenticity, and joy. Through his work and personal example, Philipp inspires others to awaken their consciousness, embrace their highest potential, and create a life that is healthy, empowered, and fulfilling.

www.ingramcontent.com/pod-product-compliance
Lightning Source LLC
Chambersburg PA
CBHW020417150626
46554CB00014B/1888